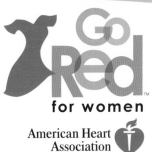

for women

American Heart
Association
Learn and Live®

LOVE YOUR HEART

50 Healthy & Delicious Recipes

5th Anniversary Edition

Publications International, Ltd.

American Heart Association Team: Linda Ball, Deborah Renza, Janice Moss, Jackie Haigney, Robin Sullivan, Barthy Gaitonde, and Michelle Overcash

Pictured on front cover: Chicken Breasts with Tomato-Kalamata Sauce (*page 47*).

Microwave Cooking: Microwave ovens vary in wattage. Use the cooking times as guidelines and check for doneness before adding more time.

Donations to the American Heart Association support its lifesaving work. For more information, call 1-800-AHA-USA1 (1-800-242-8721), contact us at americanheart.org, or write to us at 7272 Greenville Avenue, Dallas, TX 75231.

For Publications International, Ltd., business inquiries call 847-329-5841; for consumer inquiries call 847-329-5657.

Contents

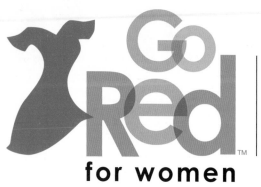

Know Red: About the Movement

Go Red For Women is the American Heart Association's nationwide movement that celebrates the energy, passion, and power we have as women to band together and wipe out heart disease.

Because of the millions of people who have already participated across the country, the color red and the red dress symbol have gained meaning and gathered momentum: They signify the ability of all women to take positive action to improve their health and live longer, stronger lives.

Heart disease is the No. 1 killer of women, but it is largely preventable. Go Red For Women empowers women by providing the knowledge and tools they need to protect their hearts.

Join the Go Red For Women movement—for your heart, for your health, for your life, and for the women you love.

Your heart is in your hands. Learn about the things you personally can do to understand your risk, take charge of your health, and get involved in heart-healthy programs.

Visit goredforwomen.org or call 1-888-MY-HEART to receive your free red dress pin and more information.

Go Red: Take It Personally!

Going Red in your own fashion is about the ways you choose to protect your heart and fight against heart disease for all women.

Right now is the time to try on some of the things you can do to Go Red:

- ♥ Take the Go Red Heart CheckUp and find out about your own heart by visiting goredforwomen.org.

- ♥ Make heart-healthy habits part of your daily life: Eat well and move more.

- ♥ Shop Go Red to support the movement by visiting shopgored.com.

- ♥ Donate your time and resources to the Go Red For Women movement.

- ♥ Host a Go Red For Women dinner party for those you love. Here are some menu ideas to get you started:

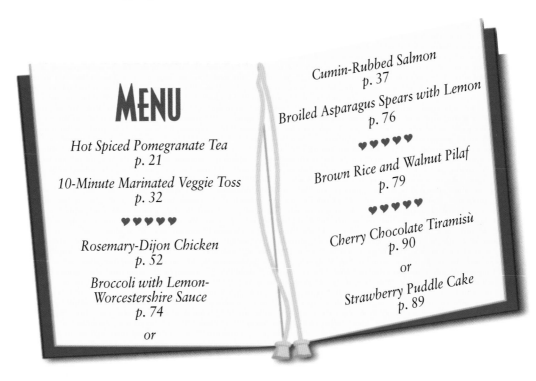

MENU

Hot Spiced Pomegranate Tea
p. 21

10-Minute Marinated Veggie Toss
p. 32

♥ ♥ ♥ ♥ ♥

Rosemary-Dijon Chicken
p. 52

Broccoli with Lemon-Worcestershire Sauce
p. 74

or

Cumin-Rubbed Salmon
p. 37

Broiled Asparagus Spears with Lemon
p. 76

♥ ♥ ♥ ♥

Brown Rice and Walnut Pilaf
p. 79

♥ ♥ ♥ ♥

Cherry Chocolate Tiramisù
p. 90

or

Strawberry Puddle Cake
p. 89

Go Red: Know Your Risks and Your Numbers

Heart disease is largely preventable because many of the risk factors are things you can control. Each factor below contributes to your overall risk of developing heart disease. If you have two or more together, your risk is even greater.

High blood pressure causes your heart to work harder than normal. Both the heart and arteries are then more prone to injury. High blood pressure increases your risk of heart attack, stroke, congestive heart failure, and buildup of plaque in arteries.

High levels of LDL cholesterol in your blood also can increase the buildup of plaque on the inner walls of your arteries. This narrows the arteries and reduces blood flow. If a plaque ruptures, it triggers a blood clot to form. If a clot forms where the plaque is, it can block blood flow or break off and travel to another part of the body. If blood flow to an artery that feeds the heart is blocked, it causes a heart attack. If the blockage occurs in an artery that feeds the brain, it causes a stroke.

Diabetes is defined by the level of glucose in your blood, which is determined by a simple blood test. Diabetes is a major risk factor for cardiovascular disease, and people with diabetes are more likely than those without it to have a heart attack or stroke.

Too much body fat—especially at your waist—means your heart has to work harder, and your risk increases for high blood pressure, high blood cholesterol, and diabetes. That's why it's so important to watch your weight and be physically active.

Consistent physical inactivity increases your risk for heart disease and stroke even more. Thirty to sixty minutes of exercise on most days of the week can actually help control high blood pressure, high blood cholesterol, diabetes, and obesity. Aerobic physical activity can also help reduce blood pressure.

Smoking and constant exposure to secondhand smoke greatly increase your risk for heart disease, stroke, and other illnesses. However, when you stop smoking—no matter how long you've smoked—your risk starts to drop. In fact, one year after quitting, your risk is cut in half. Fifteen years after quitting, your risk is similar to that of someone who has never smoked.

This chart gives you a quick overview of the numbers you and your healthcare provider will need to determine your risk of heart disease.

Factor	Goal
Blood pressure	Less than 120/80 mm Hg
Total cholesterol	Less than 200 mg/dL
LDL ("bad") cholesterol	
—No heart disease or diabetes, one or no other risk factors	Less than 160 mg/dL
—No heart disease or diabetes, two or more other risk factors	Less than 130 mg/dL
—Existing heart disease or diabetes	Less than 100 mg/dL (Some high-risk patients may have a goal of less than 70 mg/dL.)
HDL ("good") cholesterol	50 mg/dL or higher for women
Triglycerides	Less than 150 mg/dL
Blood glucose	Less than 100 mg/dL (fasting)
Waist circumference	Less than 35 inches for women
Activity level	At least 30 minutes on most, if not all, days of the week

mm Hg indicates millimeters of mercury; mg/dL, milligrams per deciliter.

You should also be aware of what level of risk for heart disease you have inherited from your family members.

Go Red: Schedule Regular Checkups

In addition to understanding the risk factors of heart disease, it's important to get early heart-health screening to help fight heart disease before it develops. Let your birthday be your reminder to schedule a health checkup every year. Find out your numbers and talk to your healthcare provider about your lifestyle and risk factors. Together, you can develop an effective plan to prevent heart disease. It's a big part of taking care of yourself and your heart.

You can also complete the Go Red Heart CheckUp. This comprehensive evaluation of your overall heart health is available online at goredforwomen.org. To fill in the questionnaire, you'll need the answers to the questions in red below.

When you visit your healthcare provider, bring along the following questions to help you remember what to ask.

Cholesterol

- ♥ What is my total cholesterol level?
- ♥ What are my HDL (good) and LDL (bad) cholesterol levels?
- ♥ What is my triglyceride level?
- ♥ What is a healthy cholesterol level?
- ♥ How often should I have my cholesterol checked?

Blood Pressure

- ♥ What is my blood pressure?
- ♥ What is my systolic number? What does it mean to my heart health?
- ♥ What is my diastolic number? What does it mean to my heart health?
- ♥ How often should I get my blood pressure checked?

Blood Glucose

- What is my fasting blood glucose (sugar level)?
- What is diabetes and how does it affect my heart health?
- What can I do to prevent developing diabetes or to manage diabetes if I already have it?

Weight

- What are my weight and height?
- What is my body mass index?
- What is a healthy weight range for me?
- Is my current weight considered healthy? Overweight? Obese?

Nutrition and Physical Activity

- How can I improve my eating habits to help my heart?
- Given my current lifestyle habits, what should I do to safely increase my activity level?
- What kind of physical activity is right for me?

Smoking

- How can I quit smoking?
- How can I avoid gaining weight after I quit smoking?

Other Risk Factors

- Does my family history put me at risk for heart disease and stroke?
- What other factors in my personal situation might affect my heart health?

Go Red: Know the Warning Signs

Not all warning signs occur with every heart attack or stroke. If you have one or more of these signs, don't wait longer than 5 minutes before calling 9-1-1 for help.

Heart Attack

Some heart attacks are sudden and intense, but most start slowly, with mild pain or discomfort.

Chest discomfort. Most heart attacks involve discomfort in the center of the chest that lasts more than a few minutes or that goes away and comes back. It can feel like uncomfortable pressure, squeezing, fullness, or pain.

Discomfort in other areas of the upper body. Symptoms can include pain or discomfort in one or both arms or in the back, neck, jaw, or stomach.

Shortness of breath. This may occur with or without chest discomfort.

Other signs. These may include breaking out in a cold sweat, nausea, or lightheadedness.

As with men, women's most common heart attack symptom is chest pain or discomfort. But women are somewhat more likely than men to experience some of the other common symptoms, particularly shortness of breath, nausea/vomiting, and back or jaw pain.

Stroke

Stroke is a medical emergency. Learn to recognize the warning signs below, because time lost is brain lost.

- Sudden numbness or weakness of the face, arm, or leg, especially on one side of the body.
- Sudden confusion, trouble speaking, or difficulty understanding.
- Sudden trouble seeing in one or both eyes.
- Sudden trouble walking, dizziness, loss of balance, or loss of coordination.
- Sudden, severe headache with no known cause.

Ask the Expert

Why should I be worried about my heart at my age? I'm only in my twenties.

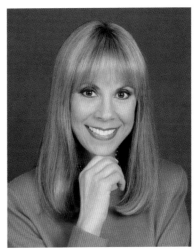

Aliza A. Lifshitz, M.D.
*American Heart Association
national spokesperson*

It's a common misconception that only older men and women suffer from heart disease or have heart attacks, but female heart attack survivors under 40 will tell you otherwise! That idea is often what keeps women from getting prompt medical attention if they experience the warning signs *(see page 12)*. Even more dangerous, most of us don't realize that the lifestyle habits we develop as young people set the stage for our health throughout our lives.

It may surprise you to know that the plaque that blocks your arteries can start forming as early as in your teens. In fact, even young children have been seen to have a buildup of plaque. Your diet and activity level have a big impact on your heart at any age.

Is heart disease really preventable?

Heart disease is largely preventable. It's never too early—or too late—to pay attention to how much saturated fat, trans fat, cholesterol, and sodium you eat. No matter what your age, you'll want to develop a sustainable eating plan that gives you all the nutrients you need and helps you manage your weight.

Similarly, establishing a routine of physical activity when you're young will help you stay active through all the stages of your life. It's also important to quit smoking, drink alcohol in moderation if at all, and get regular checkups.

These simple principles will help you avoid many of the health problems people tend to associate with aging, such as weight gain and inactivity. The steps you take now will help protect your heart and keep you healthier for life.

Recipes

Your environment, your lifestyle, and your eating habits all contribute to your overall health. In the end, it's the choices you make every day that add up to have the biggest impact. When you learn to make good choices, you and your family will enjoy the benefits for years to come.

The important thing is to be physically active and develop healthy eating habits. That means eating a wide variety of foods that promote good health.

Love Your Heart by Making Good Food Choices

Whether you are eating at home or dining out, follow the recommendations below to help protect your heart:

♥ Eat a variety of nutritious foods from all the food groups.
  ‣ Eat a diet rich in vegetables and fruits.
  ‣ Choose whole-grain, high-fiber foods.
  ‣ Eat fish, preferably fatty fish, at least twice a week.

♥ Limit foods that are high in calories but low in nutrients.
  ‣ Limit how much saturated fat, trans fat, and cholesterol you eat.
  ‣ Choose fat-free and low-fat dairy products.
  ‣ Cut back on beverages and foods with added sugars.
  ‣ Choose and prepare foods with little or no salt.
  ‣ If you drink alcohol, drink in moderation.

♥ Read nutrition facts labels and ingredients lists.

For more information on the updated American Heart Association Dietary and Lifestyle Recommendations, visit americanheart.org.

How the Recipes Are Analyzed

Each of the recipes includes a nutrition analysis. You can use these analyses to quickly determine how well a certain dish will fit into your overall eating plan. The following guidelines explain how the analyses were calculated.

- ♥ Each analysis is for a single serving; garnishes or optional ingredients are not included.

- ♥ When ingredient options are listed, the first one is analyzed. When a range of ingredients is given, the average is analyzed.

- ♥ Values for saturated, monounsaturated, and polyunsaturated fats are rounded and may not add up to the amount listed for total fat. Total fat also includes other fatty substances and glycerol.

- ♥ Meat statistics are based on cooked lean meat with all visible fat discarded.

- ♥ We use 95% fat-free ground beef for analysis.

- ♥ When analyzing recipes that call for alcohol, we estimate that most of the alcohol calories evaporate during cooking.

- ♥ We use the abbreviations "g" for gram and "mg" for milligram.

Appetizers, Snacks & Beverages

ALMOND SNACK MIX

SERVES 4; ½ cup per serving

⅓ cup whole unsalted almonds

⅔ cup multibran or whole-grain cereal squares

½ cup low-fat granola cereal without raisins

¼ cup dried apricot halves, cut into strips, or golden raisins

¼ cup sweetened dried cranberries

Preheat the oven to 350°F. Spread the almonds in a single layer on an ungreased baking sheet. Bake for 5 to 10 minutes, or until lightly toasted, stirring once or twice to ensure even baking. Transfer to a plate to cool completely.

Meanwhile, in a large bowl, stir together the remaining ingredients. Stir in the cooled almonds.

Nutrients per Serving: Calories 174, Total Fat 6.5 g, Saturated Fat 0.5 g, Polyunsaturated Fat 1.5 g, Monounsaturated Fat 4.0 g, Cholesterol 0 mg, Sodium 72 mg, Carbohydrates 29 g, Fiber 5 g, Sugars 14 g, Protein 4 g

Dietary Exchanges: 1 starch, 1 fruit, 1 fat

Cook's Tip

If all the snack mix isn't likely to be eaten on the day you make it, we recommend using the golden raisins. The moisture of the dried apricots may cause the cereal to lose its crispness over time. Be sure the almonds are completely cooled when you add them to the mix; otherwise, they will make it soggy.

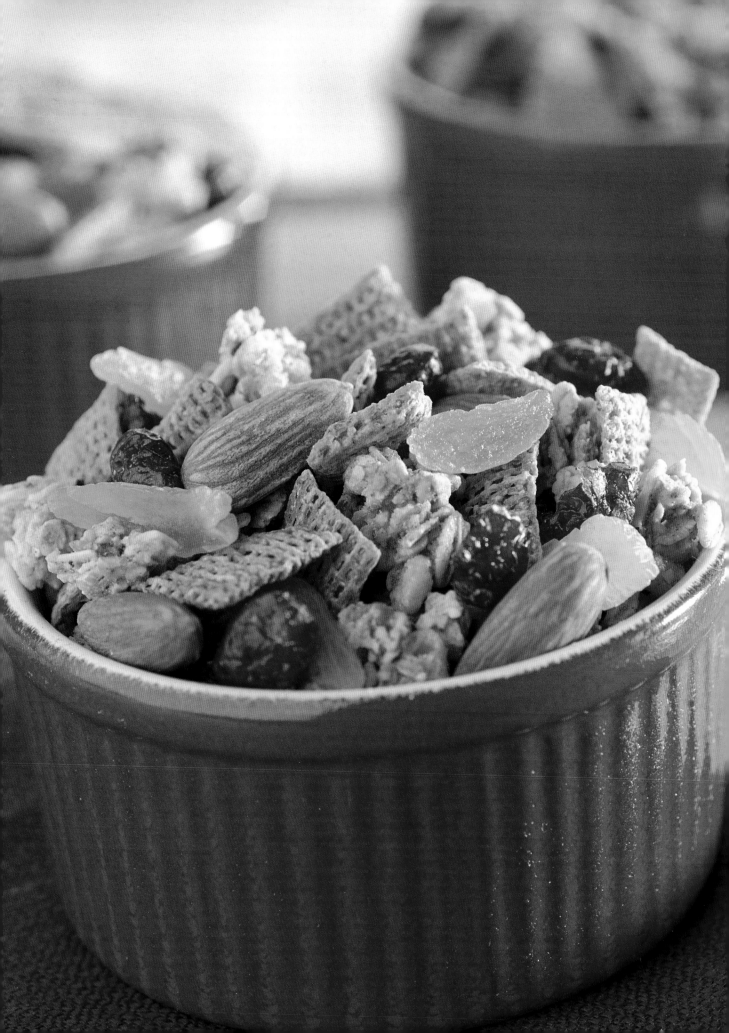

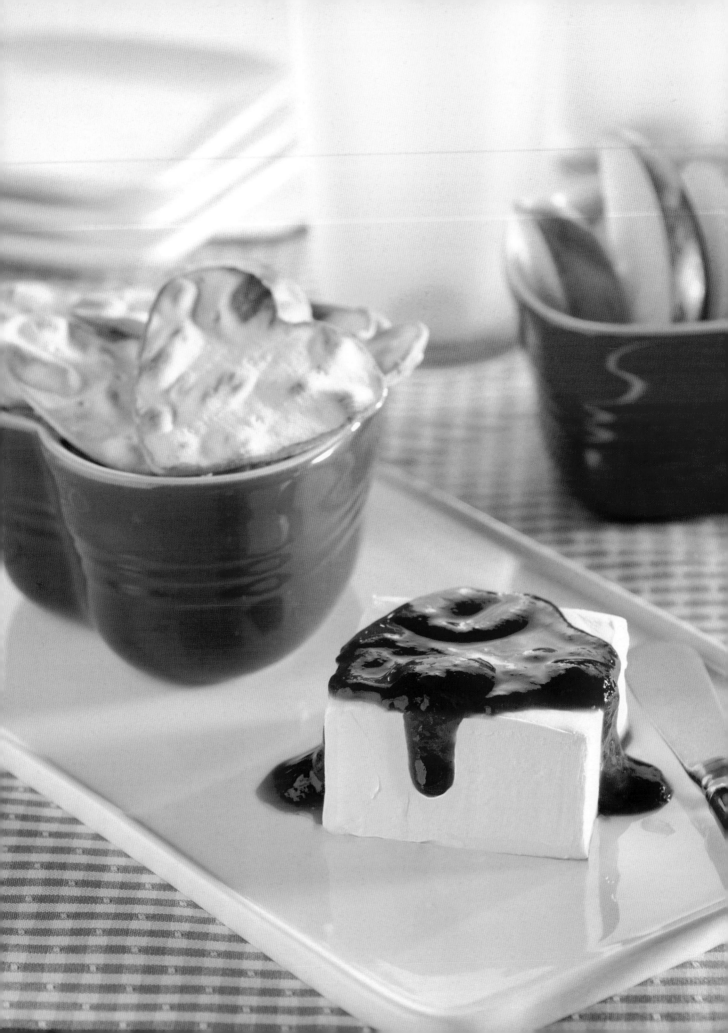

RASPBERRY-PEPPER JELLY OVER CREAM CHEESE

SERVES 8; 1 tablespoon cream cheese,
1½ teaspoons jelly mixture, and 3 crackers or 3 slices of fruit per serving

¼ cup all-fruit seedless raspberry spread

½ teaspoon balsamic vinegar

⅛ teaspoon ground cinnamon

⅛ teaspoon crushed red pepper flakes

4 ounces fat-free or light cream cheese

24 fat-free or low-fat, low-sodium crackers or 3 medium red apples or red-skinned pears, each cut into 8 slices

In a small microwaveable bowl, stir together the fruit spread, vinegar, cinnamon, and red pepper flakes. Heat in a microwave on 100 percent power (high) for 15 seconds, or until melted. Stir. Let cool completely.

Put the cream cheese on a plate. Spoon the raspberry mixture on top. Serve with the crackers or fruit.

WITH CRACKERS — Nutrients per Serving: Calories 69, Total Fat 0.0 g, Saturated Fat 0.0 g, Polyunsaturated Fat 0.0 g, Monounsaturated Fat 0.0 g, Cholesterol 3 mg, Sodium 124 mg, Carbohydrates 13 g, Fiber 0 g, Sugars 5 g, Protein 3 g
Dietary Exchanges: 1 starch

WITH FRUIT — Nutrients per Serving: Calories 62, Total Fat 0.0 g, Saturated Fat 0.0 g, Polyunsaturated Fat 0.0 g, Monounsaturated Fat 0.0 g, Cholesterol 3 mg, Sodium 71 mg, Carbohydrates 13 g, Fiber 1 g, Sugars 10 g, Protein 2 g
Dietary Exchanges: 1 fruit

BLACK BEAN DIP WITH FRESH LIME

SERVES 6; 2 tablespoons dip per serving

½ 15-ounce can no-salt-added black beans, rinsed and drained
¼ cup snipped fresh cilantro
2 tablespoons chopped red onion
2 tablespoons fresh lime juice
1 tablespoon water
1 tablespoon fat-free or light mayonnaise
1½ teaspoons olive oil
¼ teaspoon ground cumin
¼ teaspoon salt
¼ teaspoon red hot-pepper sauce, or to taste
1 tablespoon water (optional)

In a food processor or blender, process all the ingredients except the optional 1 tablespoon water until smooth. For a thinner consistency, gradually add the remaining water until the dip is the desired consistency.

Nutrients per Serving: Calories 45, Total Fat 1.0 g, Saturated Fat 0.0 g, Polyunsaturated Fat 0.0 g, Monounsaturated Fat 1.0 g, Cholesterol 0 mg, Sodium 119 mg, Carbohydrates 7 g, Fiber 2 g, Sugars 2 g, Protein 2 g

Dietary Exchanges: ½ starch

HOT SPICED POMEGRANATE TEA

SERVES 4; 1 cup per serving

1   15.2-ounce bottle pomegranate juice
2½ cups water
¼   cup sugar
1   medium orange, cut crosswise into 8 slices
4   cinnamon sticks, each about 3 inches long
6   whole cloves
2   unflavored tea bags
½   medium lemon, cut crosswise into 4 slices
2   orange slices, halved (optional)

In a medium saucepan, stir together the pomegranate juice, water, sugar, 8 orange slices, cinnamon sticks, and cloves. Bring to a boil over high heat. Reduce the heat and simmer for 8 minutes, or until the flavors blend. Remove from the heat.

Add the tea bags and lemon slices. Steep for 2 minutes. Pour the mixture through a sieve into a teapot, retaining the cinnamon sticks. Pour the tea into cups or mugs. Put a cinnamon stick and halved orange slice in each.

Nutrients per Serving:
Calories 115, Total Fat 0.0 g, Saturated Fat 0.0 g, Polyunsaturated Fat 0.0 g, Monounsaturated Fat 0.0 g, Cholesterol 0 mg, Sodium 17 mg, Carbohydrates 29 g, Fiber 0 g, Sugars 29 g, Protein 1 g
Dietary Exchanges: 1 fruit, 1 other carbohydrate

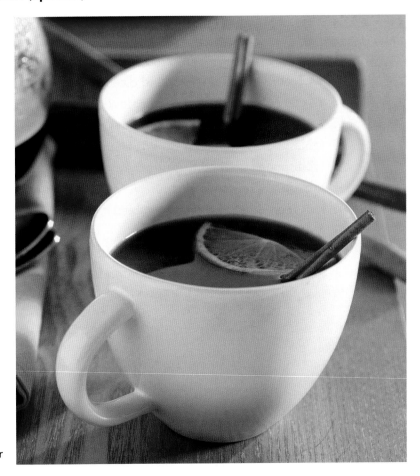

Soups

RUSTIC ITALIAN TOMATO SOUP

SERVES 4; 1 cup per serving

1 16-ounce package frozen mixed bell pepper strips (may be labeled stir-fry mix)
1 14.5-ounce can no-salt-added diced tomatoes, undrained
1 14- or 14.5-ounce can fat-free, low-sodium chicken broth
½ 15.5-ounce can no-salt-added navy beans, rinsed and drained
3 tablespoons chopped fresh basil leaves
2 tablespoons snipped fresh parsley
1 tablespoon balsamic vinegar
½ teaspoon dried oregano, crumbled
1 medium garlic clove, minced
⅛ to ¼ teaspoon crushed red pepper flakes
1 tablespoon olive oil (extra-virgin preferred)
¼ teaspoon salt

In a food processor or blender, process the bell peppers, undrained tomatoes, broth, beans, basil, parsley, vinegar, oregano, garlic, and red pepper flakes until slightly chunky or smooth. Pour into a large saucepan. Bring to a boil over high heat. Reduce the heat and simmer, covered, for 20 minutes, or until the flavors are blended. Remove from the heat. Stir in the oil and salt. Ladle into soup bowls.

Nutrients per Serving: Calories 136, Total Fat 3.5 g, Saturated Fat 0.5 g, Polyunsaturated Fat 0.5 g, Monounsaturated Fat 2.5 g, Cholesterol 0 mg, Sodium 215 mg, Carbohydrates 22 g, Fiber 5 g, Sugars 12 g, Protein 5 g
Dietary Exchanges: ½ starch, 3 vegetable, ½ fat

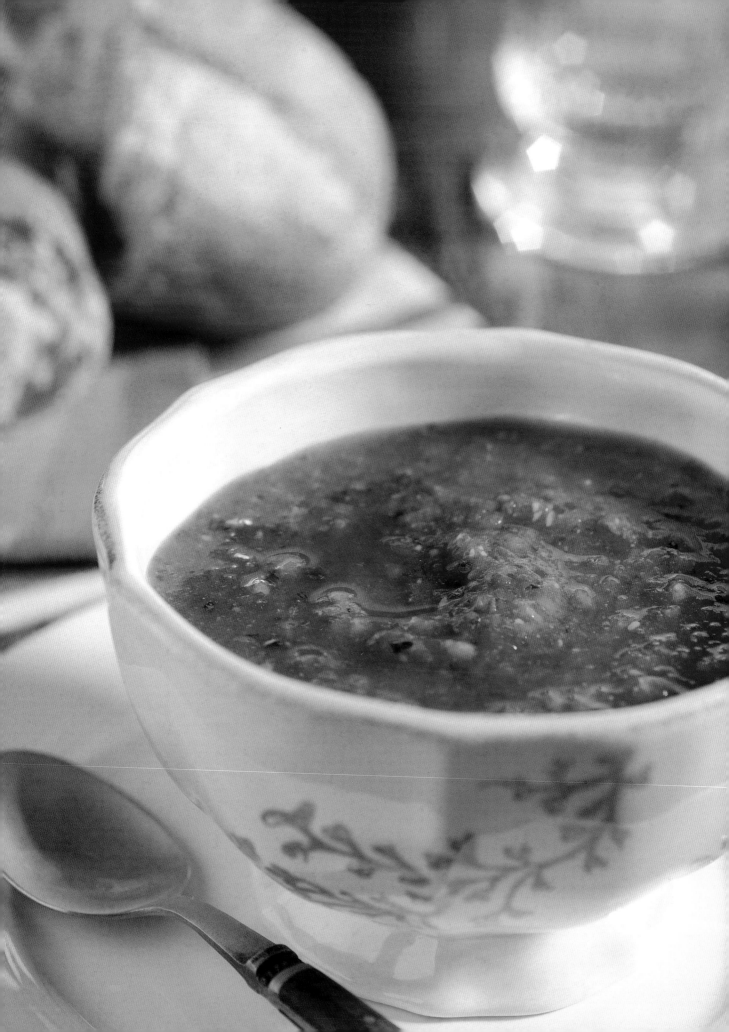

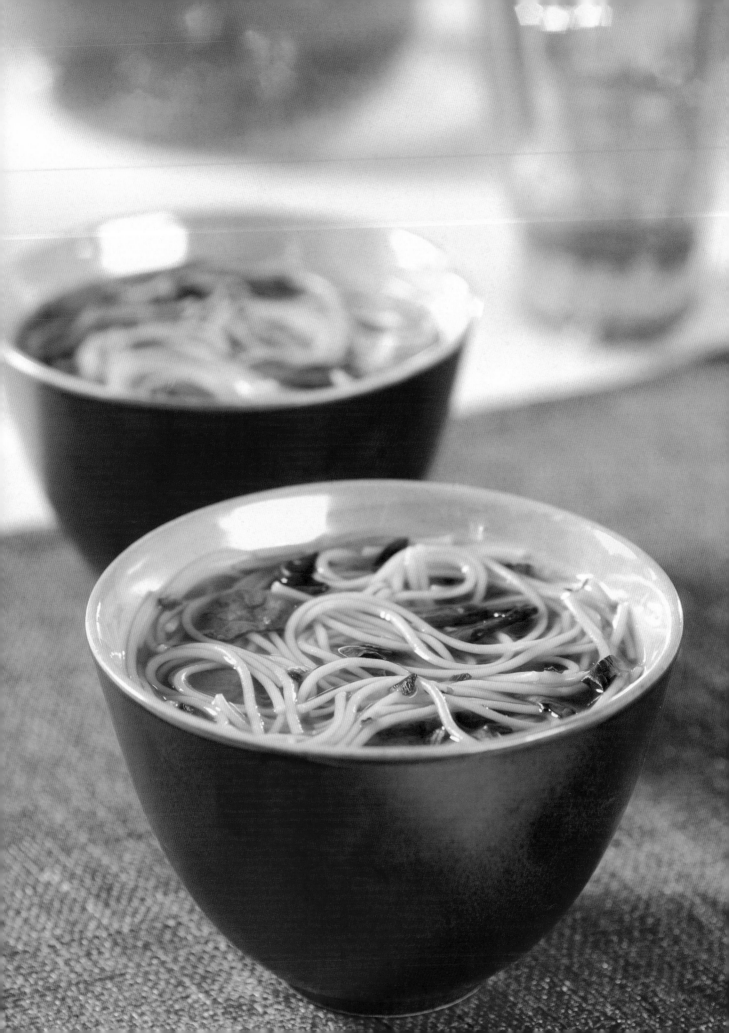

SPINACH NOODLE BOWL WITH BASIL AND GINGER

SERVES 4; 1 cup per serving

   2 14-ounce cans fat-free, low-sodium chicken broth
 1½ ounces dried angel hair pasta, broken into 2-inch pieces, if desired
  ⅛ teaspoon crushed red pepper flakes (optional)
   1 cup baby spinach leaves, coarsely chopped
  ¼ cup chopped fresh basil leaves
   2 teaspoons grated peeled gingerroot

In a medium saucepan, bring the broth to a boil over high heat. Stir in the pasta and red pepper flakes. Return to a boil. Reduce the heat and simmer, covered, for 6 minutes, or until the pasta is just tender. Remove from the heat.

Stir in the remaining ingredients. Let stand for 2 minutes to absorb flavors.

Nutrients per Serving: Calories 51, Total Fat 0.0 g, Saturated Fat 0.0 g, Polyunsaturated Fat 0.0 g, Monounsaturated Fat 0.0 g, Cholesterol 0 mg, Sodium 56 mg, Carbohydrates 9 g, Fiber 1 g, Sugars 1 g, Protein 3 g

Dietary Exchanges: ½ starch

CHILLED STRAWBERRY-RASPBERRY SOUP

SERVES 5; 1 cup per serving

2 cups whole fresh strawberries

1 cup fresh or frozen unsweetened raspberries

1 cup fat-free or low-fat plain yogurt

2 tablespoons sugar

2 tablespoons honey

½ teaspoon grated orange zest

1¾ cups fresh orange juice

½ teaspoon vanilla extract

5 whole strawberries with caps (optional)

5 orange zest curls (optional)

In a food processor or blender, process all the ingredients except the strawberries with caps and the orange zest until smooth. Refrigerate, covered, to chill if desired.

Make strawberry fans for a garnish by thinly slicing each strawberry lengthwise to, but not all the way through, the cap. Press down gently on the cap end to separate the slices into a fan.

To serve, ladle the soup into bowls. Place a curl of orange zest on top of, and a strawberry fan beside, each serving.

Nutrients per Serving:
Calories 142, Total Fat 0.5 g, Saturated Fat 0.0 g, Polyunsaturated Fat 0.0 g, Monounsaturated Fat 0.0 g, Cholesterol 1 mg, Sodium 40 mg, Carbohydrates 32 g, Fiber 3 g, Sugars 28 g, Protein 4 g

Dietary Exchanges: 1 fruit, 1 other carbohydrate, ½ skim milk

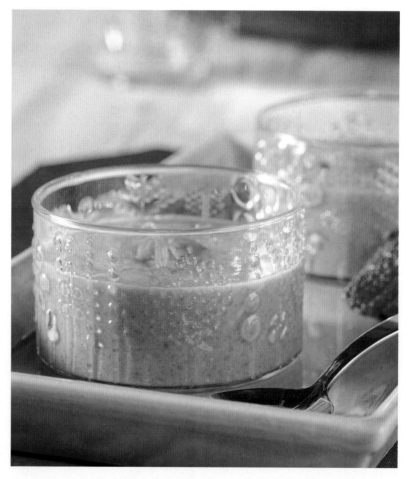

CHICKEN AND ROTINI SOUP

SERVES 4; 1¼ cups per serving

Vegetable oil spray

8   ounces boneless, skinless chicken breasts, all visible fat discarded, cut into ½-inch pieces

2   14- or 14.5-ounce cans fat-free, low-sodium chicken broth

1   medium red bell pepper, thinly sliced and cut into 2-inch strips

1   medium green bell pepper, thinly sliced and cut into 2-inch strips

⅛   teaspoon crushed red pepper flakes

4   ounces dried rotini

2   tablespoons fresh basil leaves, chopped

½   teaspoon salt

⅛   teaspoon pepper

¼   cup grated or shredded Parmesan cheese

Lightly spray a large saucepan with vegetable oil spray. Heat over medium heat. Cook the chicken for 2 minutes, or until beginning to lightly brown, stirring frequently. (The chicken will still be slightly pink in the center.) Stir in the broth, bell peppers, and pepper flakes. Increase the heat to high and bring to a boil. Stir. Reduce the heat and simmer for 3 minutes, or until the bell peppers are tender-crisp.

Increase the heat to high and return to a boil. Stir in the rotini. Reduce the heat and simmer for 6 minutes, or until just tender. Stir in the basil, salt, and pepper. Ladle into soup bowls. Sprinkle with the Parmesan.

Nutrients per Serving: Calories 211, Total Fat 2.5 g, Saturated Fat 1.0 g, Polyunsaturated Fat 0.5 g, Monounsaturated Fat 0.5 g, Cholesterol 37 mg, Sodium 465 mg, Carbohydrates 25 g, Fiber 2 g, Sugars 3 g, Protein 21 g

Dietary Exchanges: 1½ starch, 1 vegetable, 2 very lean meat

Salads

PEAR AND SPINACH SALAD WITH CITRUS-GINGER DRESSING

SERVES 4; 2 cups salad and 2 tablespoons dressing per serving

4 cups packed spinach leaves (about 4 ounces)
2 firm pears, cut into medium slices
¼ cup thinly sliced red onion

Dressing

¼ cup frozen white grape juice concentrate
2 teaspoons sugar
1 teaspoon grated peeled gingerroot
½ teaspoon grated orange zest
½ teaspoon grated lemon zest
3 tablespoons fresh lemon juice
⅛ teaspoon crushed red pepper flakes

Arrange the spinach on a serving platter. Place the pears and onion on the spinach.

In a small jar with a tight-fitting lid, combine the dressing ingredients. Shake vigorously until well blended. Pour over the salad.

Nutrients per Serving: Calories 104, Total Fat 0.5 g, Saturated Fat 0.0 g, Polyunsaturated Fat 0.0 g, Monounsaturated Fat 0.0 g, Cholesterol 0 mg, Sodium 26 mg, Carbohydrates 26 g, Fiber 3 g, Sugars 19 g, Protein 2 g

Dietary Exchanges: 1½ fruit

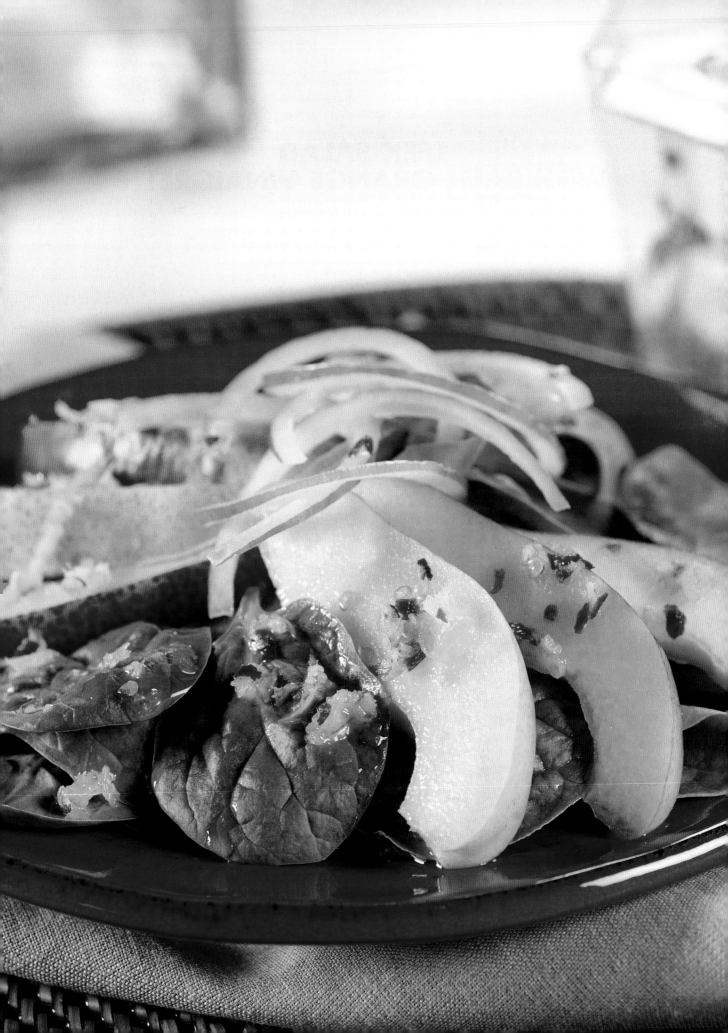

LEEK SALAD
WITH BASIL-ORANGE VINAIGRETTE

SERVES 4; ⅓ cup per serving

  2 to 3 medium leeks

  ½ medium red, yellow, or green bell pepper

Basil-Orange Vinaigrette

  3 tablespoons tarragon vinegar or white wine vinegar

  ½ teaspoon grated orange zest

  2 tablespoons fresh orange juice

  1 tablespoon olive (extra-virgin preferred), canola, or corn oil

  1 tablespoon finely chopped fresh basil or ½ teaspoon dried basil, crumbled

  1 teaspoon Dijon mustard

• • •

  4 large lettuce leaves, such as red leaf

Remove the root ends of the leeks right where they join the white bulbs. Remove all but about 1 inch of the green tops. Slice the leeks about ½ inch thick. Put the pieces in a large bowl of cool water, rinsing thoroughly to remove all traces of dirt and grit. In a small saucepan, cook the leeks in a small amount of boiling water for 5 minutes. Pour into a colander and drain well. Let cool.

Meanwhile, chop the bell pepper and put in a medium bowl. When the leeks are cool, toss them with the bell pepper.

Put the dressing ingredients in a screw-top jar. Cover and shake until well combined. Pour over the leek mixture, tossing to coat. Cover and chill for 1 to 24 hours, tossing occasionally. Serve on the lettuce leaves.

Nutrients per Serving: Calories 75, Total Fat 3.5 g, Saturated Fat 0.5 g, Polyunsaturated Fat 0.5 g, Monounsaturated Fat 2.5 g, Cholesterol 0 mg, Sodium 42 mg, Carbohydrates 10 g, Fiber 2 g, Sugars 3 g, Protein 1 g

Dietary Exchanges: 2 vegetable, 1 fat

TUNA-TOPPED VEGGIE AND PASTA SALAD

SERVES 4; 1½ cups per serving

    6 ounces dried tricolor rotini
    1 14-ounce can quartered artichoke hearts, rinsed and well drained
    1 cup quartered grape tomatoes or cherry tomatoes (about 5 ounces)
    ½ medium green bell pepper, chopped
    ⅓ cup finely chopped red onion
    2 tablespoons chopped fresh basil leaves
    2 tablespoons cider vinegar
    2 tablespoons olive oil (extra-virgin preferred)
    1 medium garlic clove, minced
    ¼ teaspoon salt
    1 7-ounce vacuum-sealed pouch light tuna

Prepare the pasta using the package directions, omitting the salt and oil. Drain in a colander. Run under cold water to cool quickly. Drain well. Transfer to a large bowl.

Add the remaining ingredients except the tuna. Toss gently. Spoon onto plates. Sprinkle with the tuna. Do not stir.

Nutrients per Serving: Calories 316, Total Fat 8.0 g, Saturated Fat 1.0 g, Polyunsaturated Fat 1.5 g, Monounsaturated Fat 5.0 g, Cholesterol 27 mg, Sodium 539 mg, Carbohydrates 41 g, Fiber 3 g, Sugars 5 g, Protein 19 g

Dietary Exchanges: 2 starch, 2 vegetable, 2 lean meat

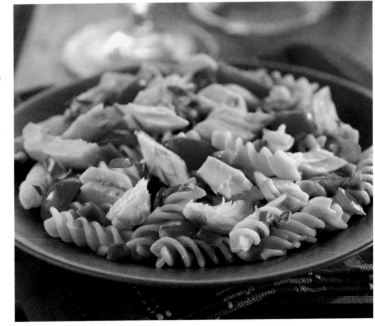

10-MINUTE MARINATED VEGGIE TOSS

SERVES 6; ½ cup per serving

1	14-ounce can quartered artichoke hearts, rinsed and well drained
¼	medium red bell pepper, thinly sliced
¼	cup thinly sliced red onion
¼	cup packed fresh baby spinach leaves, torn if desired
9	small black olives, halved
2	teaspoons cider vinegar
1½	teaspoons sugar
1	teaspoon olive oil
1	medium garlic clove, minced

In a medium bowl, stir together all the ingredients. Let stand for 10 minutes. For peak flavors, serve immediately after the standing time.

Nutrients per Serving: Calories 35, Total Fat 1.5 g, Saturated Fat 0.0 g, Polyunsaturated Fat 0.0 g, Monounsaturated Fat 1.0 g, Cholesterol 0 mg, Sodium 151 mg, Carbohydrates 5 g, Fiber 1 g, Sugars 2 g, Protein 1 g
Dietary Exchanges: 1 vegetable

Cook's Tip

For additional nutrients and color, spoon the salad onto a bed of spinach leaves.

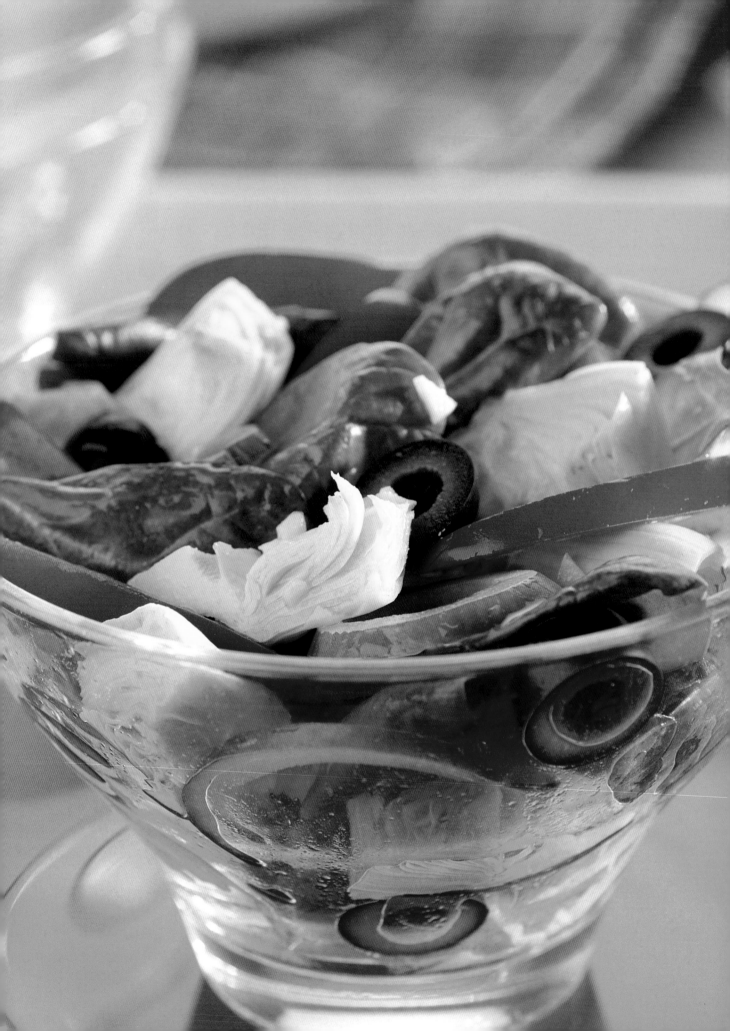

Seafood

TILAPIA WITH SMOKY-PEPPER SAUCE

SERVES 4; 3 ounces fish and ⅓ cup sauce per serving

- 4 tilapia or other mild, thin fish fillets (about 4 ounces each)
- ½ teaspoon paprika
- ¼ teaspoon pepper
- 1 teaspoon canola or olive oil
- ¾ cup finely chopped bottled roasted red bell peppers
- ½ cup mild picante sauce (lowest sodium available)
- ½ to 1 chipotle pepper canned in adobo sauce, finely chopped and mashed with a fork
- 2 teaspoons olive oil
- ¼ teaspoon minced garlic

Rinse the fish and pat dry with paper towels. Sprinkle the paprika and pepper on both sides of the fish. In a large nonstick skillet, heat the oil over medium heat, swirling to coat the bottom. Cook the fish for 3 minutes on each side, or until it flakes easily when tested with a fork. Transfer the fish to plates.

Meanwhile, in a small microwaveable bowl, stir together the remaining ingredients. Cover the bowl with plastic wrap. Microwave on 100 percent power (high) for 2 minutes, or until thoroughly heated. Spoon over the cooked fish.

Nutrients per Serving: Calories 151, Total Fat 5.5 g, Saturated Fat 1.0 g, Polyunsaturated Fat 1.0 g, Monounsaturated Fat 3.0 g, Cholesterol 57 mg, Sodium 329 mg, Carbohydrates 3 g, Fiber 0 g, Sugars 0 g, Protein 23 g

Dietary Exchanges: 3 lean meat

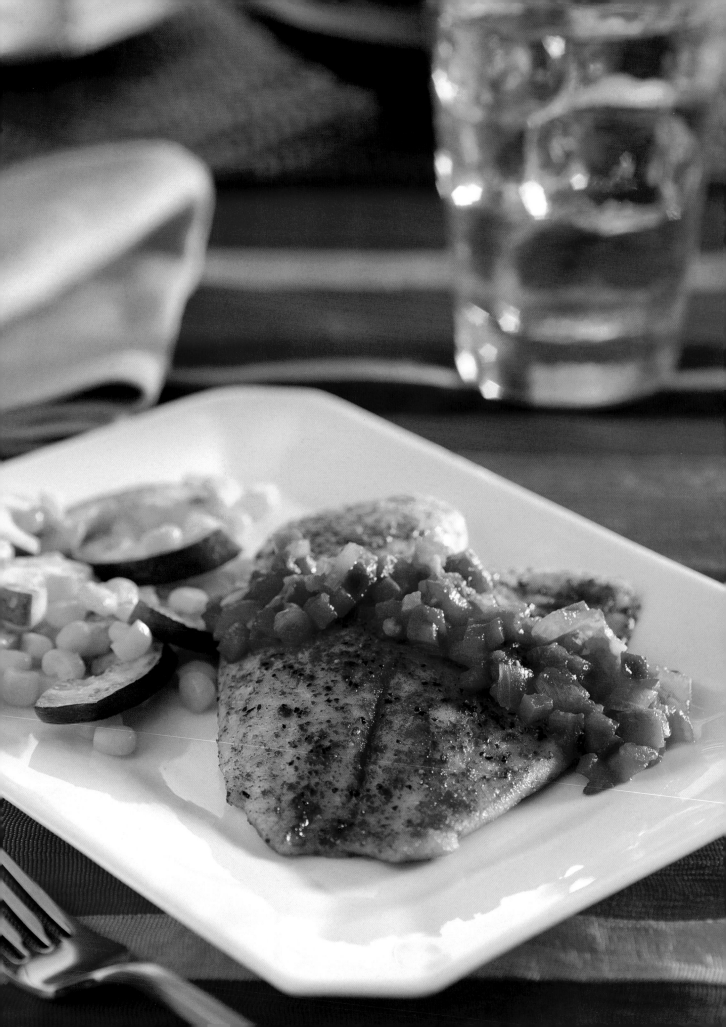

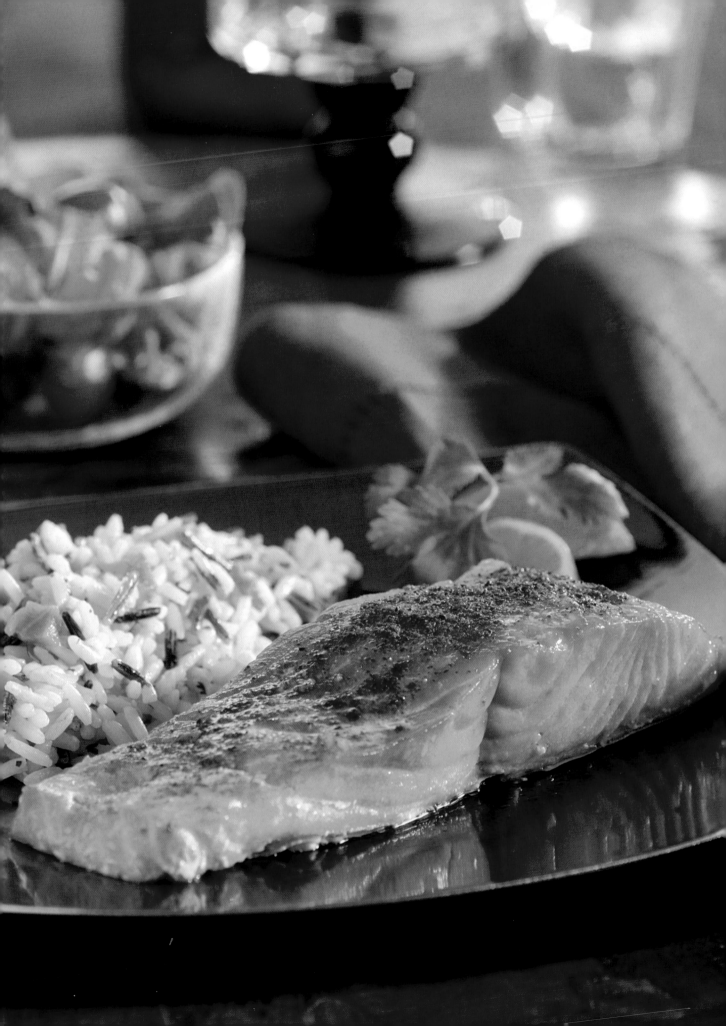

CUMIN-RUBBED SALMON

SERVES 4; 3 ounces fish per serving

Vegetable oil spray

4 salmon fillets (about 4 ounces each)

¼ teaspoon ground cumin

¼ teaspoon chili powder

¼ teaspoon salt

¼ teaspoon paprika

Preheat the oven to 350°F. Line a baking sheet with aluminum foil and lightly spray with vegetable oil spray.

Rinse the fish and pat dry with paper towels. Place the fish with the smooth side up in a single layer on the baking sheet.

In a small bowl, stir together the remaining ingredients. Sprinkle on top of the fish. Using your fingertips, gently press the mixture into the fish so it will adhere.

Bake for 18 to 20 minutes, or until the fish flakes easily when tested with a fork.

Nutrients per Serving: Calories 145, Total Fat 4.5 g, Saturated Fat 0.5 g, Polyunsaturated Fat 1.5 g, Monounsaturated Fat 1.0 g, Cholesterol 65 mg, Sodium 230 mg, Carbohydrates 0 g, Fiber 0 g, Sugars 0 g, Protein 25 g

Dietary Exchanges: 3 lean meat

GREEK SHRIMP

SERVES 4; 1⅓ cups per serving

1 pound peeled raw medium shrimp (1 to 1¼ pounds with tails), rinsed and patted dry with paper towels

1 tablespoon plus 1½ teaspoons dried Greek seasoning blend

⅛ teaspoon cayenne

1 large tomato, seeded and diced

½ cup chopped green onion

¼ cup snipped fresh parsley

1 tablespoon grated lemon zest

2 tablespoons fresh lemon juice

2 tablespoons capers, rinsed and drained

1 tablespoon plus 1½ teaspoons olive oil (extra-virgin preferred)

¼ teaspoon salt

2 cups hot cooked brown rice

Heat a large nonstick skillet over medium-high heat. Cook the shrimp, seasoning blend, and cayenne for 5 minutes, or until the shrimp turn pink on the outside and opaque in the center, stirring frequently. Stir in the remaining ingredients. Cook for 1 minute, or until heated through.

To serve, spoon the rice onto plates. Spoon the shrimp mixture over the rice.

Nutrients per Serving: Calories 191, Total Fat 6.5 g, Saturated Fat 1.0 g, Polyunsaturated Fat 1.0 g, Monounsaturated Fat 4.0 g, Cholesterol 168 mg, Sodium 559 mg, Carbohydrates 13 g, Fiber 2 g, Sugars 2 g, Protein 20 g

Dietary Exchanges: ½ starch, 1 vegetable, 3 lean meat

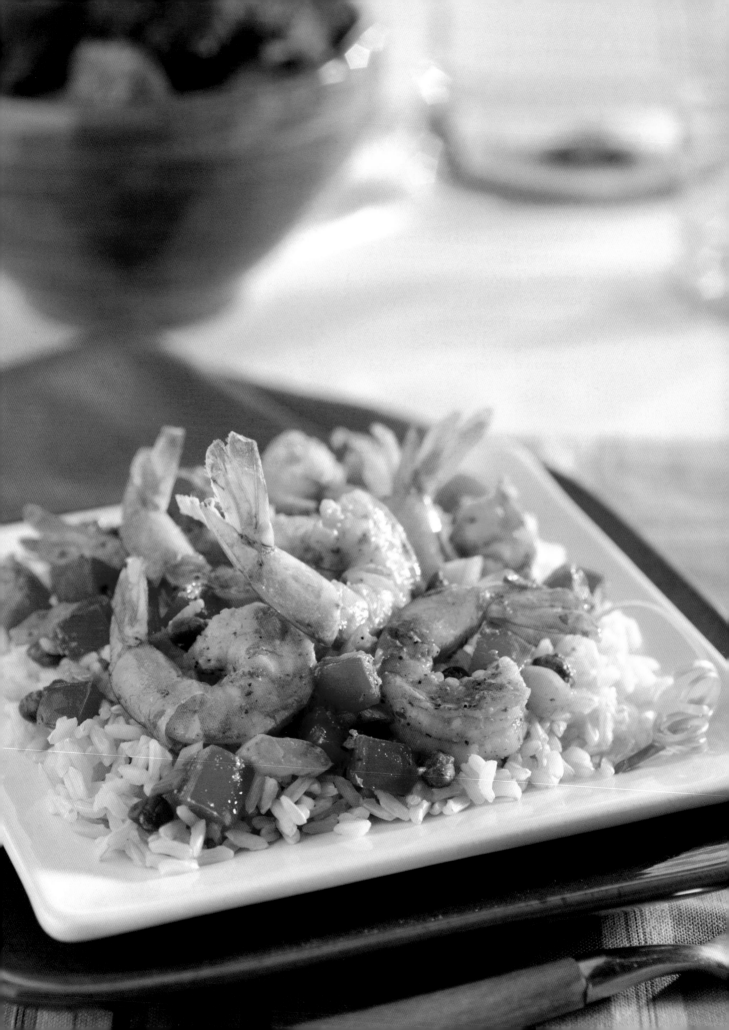

BROILED HALIBUT WITH HERBED MUSTARD

SERVES 4; 3 ounces fish per serving

Vegetable oil spray
4 halibut or other mild fish fillets (about 4 ounces each)
¼ teaspoon salt
¼ teaspoon pepper
3 tablespoons light tub margarine
1 tablespoon Dijon mustard
1 teaspoon grated lemon zest
½ teaspoon dried oregano, crumbled

Preheat the broiler. Line a broiler pan with aluminum foil. Lightly spray the foil with vegetable oil spray.

Rinse the fish and pat dry with paper towels. Put the fish on the foil. Sprinkle the fish with the salt and pepper. Lightly spray the fish with vegetable oil spray.

Broil the fish (on one side only) about 4 inches from the heat for 6 minutes (4 to 6 minutes for thinner fish), or until it flakes easily when tested with a fork. Transfer the fish to a serving platter.

Meanwhile, in a small bowl, stir together the remaining ingredients.

To serve, spoon the margarine mixture over the fish.

Nutrients per Serving: Calories 161, Total Fat 6.5 g, Saturated Fat 0.5 g, Polyunsaturated Fat 1.5 g, Monounsaturated Fat 2.5 g, Cholesterol 36 mg, Sodium 351 mg, Carbohydrates 1 g, Fiber 0 g, Sugars 0 g, Protein 24 g
Dietary Exchanges: 3 lean meat

Cook's Tip

Lightly spraying vegetable oil spray on the fish helps keep the fish moist as it cooks.

MEDITERRANEAN FISH

SERVES 4; 3 ounces fish and 2 tablespoons tomato mixture per serving

Vegetable oil spray

4 dry-packed sun-dried tomato halves, finely chopped

2 tablespoons water

8 kalamata olives, finely chopped

2 tablespoons diced pimiento

2 tablespoons finely snipped fresh parsley

1 tablespoon chopped fresh basil leaves

1 teaspoon olive oil

4 mild, thin fish fillets, such as snapper (about 4 ounces each)

¼ teaspoon paprika

⅛ teaspoon cayenne

⅛ teaspoon salt

Preheat the oven to 400°F. Line a baking sheet with aluminum foil and lightly spray with vegetable oil spray.

In a small microwaveable bowl, stir together the tomatoes and water. Cover with plastic wrap. Microwave on 100 percent power (high) for 30 seconds, or until the water is very hot. Let stand for 5 minutes, or until the tomatoes are soft. Drain well. Return the tomatoes to the bowl. Stir in the olives, pimiento, parsley, basil, and oil.

Rinse the fish and pat dry with paper towels. Place the fish in a single layer on the baking sheet. Sprinkle with the paprika, cayenne, and salt.

Bake for 10 minutes, or until the fish flakes easily when tested with a fork. Transfer the fish to a serving plate. Spoon the tomato mixture on top.

Nutrients per Serving: Calories 152, Total Fat 4.5 g, Saturated Fat 0.5 g, Polyunsaturated Fat 1.0 g, Monounsaturated Fat 2.5 g, Cholesterol 40 mg, Sodium 246 mg, Carbohydrates 3 g, Fiber 1 g, Sugars 1 g, Protein 23 g

Dietary Exchanges: 3 lean meat

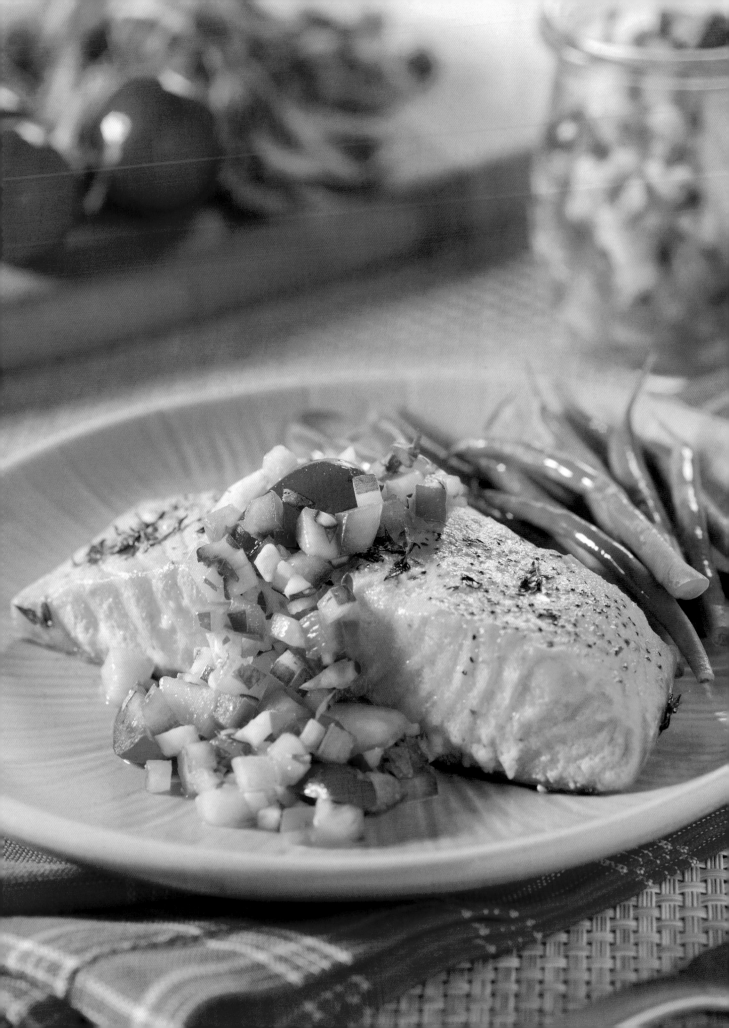

THYME-ROASTED SALMON WITH CRUNCHY VEGGIE SALSA

SERVES 4; 3 ounces fish and ¼ cup salsa per serving

Salsa

½ medium cucumber (about 3 ounces), peeled, seeded, and chopped

¼ cup quartered or chopped grape tomatoes

½ medium green bell pepper, chopped

¼ cup finely chopped radishes

2 tablespoons snipped fresh cilantro

2 tablespoons finely chopped red onion

1 teaspoon grated lime zest

2 tablespoons fresh lime juice

1 teaspoon olive oil (extra-virgin preferred)

¼ teaspoon salt

• • •

Vegetable oil spray

4 salmon fillets (about 4 ounces each)

1 teaspoon dried thyme, crumbled

¼ teaspoon salt

¼ teaspoon coarsely ground black pepper

Preheat the oven to 350°F.

In a medium bowl, gently stir together the salsa ingredients. Set aside.

Line a baking sheet with aluminum foil. Lightly spray with vegetable oil spray.

Rinse the fish and pat dry with paper towels. Put the fish on the foil. Sprinkle the fish with the thyme, salt, and pepper.

Bake for 20 minutes, or until the fish flakes easily when tested with a fork.

To serve, transfer the fish to plates. Spoon the salsa and its accumulated juices over or beside the fish.

Nutrients per Serving: Calories 156, Total Fat 5.0 g, Saturated Fat 1.0 g, Polyunsaturated Fat 1.5 g, Monounsaturated Fat 2.0 g, Cholesterol 59 mg, Sodium 372 mg, Carbohydrates 3 g, Fiber 1 g, Sugars 1 g, Protein 23 g

Dietary Exchanges: 3 lean meat

Poultry

PICANTE CHICKEN

SERVES 4; 3 ounces chicken, ½ cup rice, and 1 tablespoon sauce per serving

    Vegetable oil spray
- 4 boneless, skinless chicken breast halves (about 4 ounces each), all visible fat discarded
- ¼ to ½ teaspoon ground cumin
- 2 teaspoons olive oil
- ¼ cup mild picante sauce (lowest sodium available)
- 1 cup uncooked instant brown rice
- ¼ teaspoon ground turmeric (optional)
- ¼ teaspoon salt
- 2 tablespoons fat-free or light sour cream
- 2 tablespoons snipped fresh cilantro

Preheat the oven to 350°F.

Lightly spray an 11×7×2-inch baking dish with vegetable oil spray. Put the chicken in the baking dish. Sprinkle with the cumin, drizzle with the oil, and spoon the picante sauce on top. Using the back of a spoon, spread the sauce evenly over the chicken.

Bake for 25 minutes, or until the chicken is no longer pink in the center.

Meanwhile, in a small saucepan, prepare the rice according to the package directions, omitting the salt and margarine and adding the turmeric. Stir in the salt.

To serve, spoon the rice onto plates. Place the chicken beside the rice. Spoon the sauce over all. Top the chicken with the sour cream and cilantro.

Nutrients per Serving: Calories 245, Total Fat 4.5 g, Saturated Fat 0.5 g, Polyunsaturated Fat 1.0 g, Monounsaturated Fat 2.5 g, Cholesterol 67 mg, Sodium 296 mg, Carbohydrates 20 g, Fiber 1 g, Sugars 1 g, Protein 29 g

Dietary Exchanges: 1½ starch, 3 very lean meat

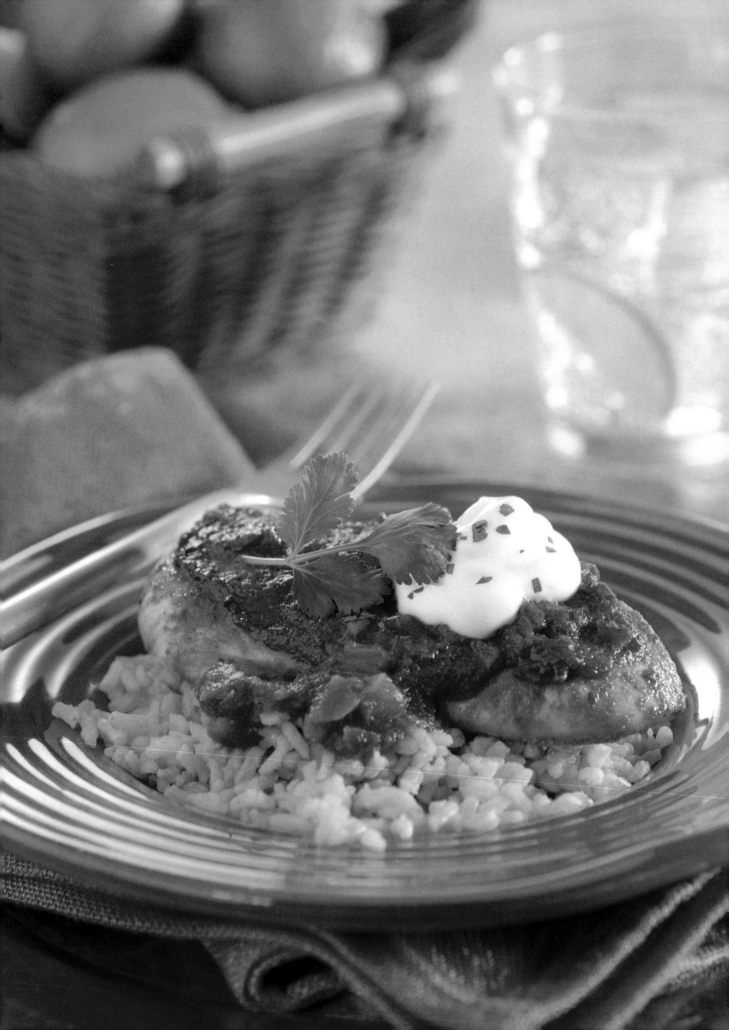

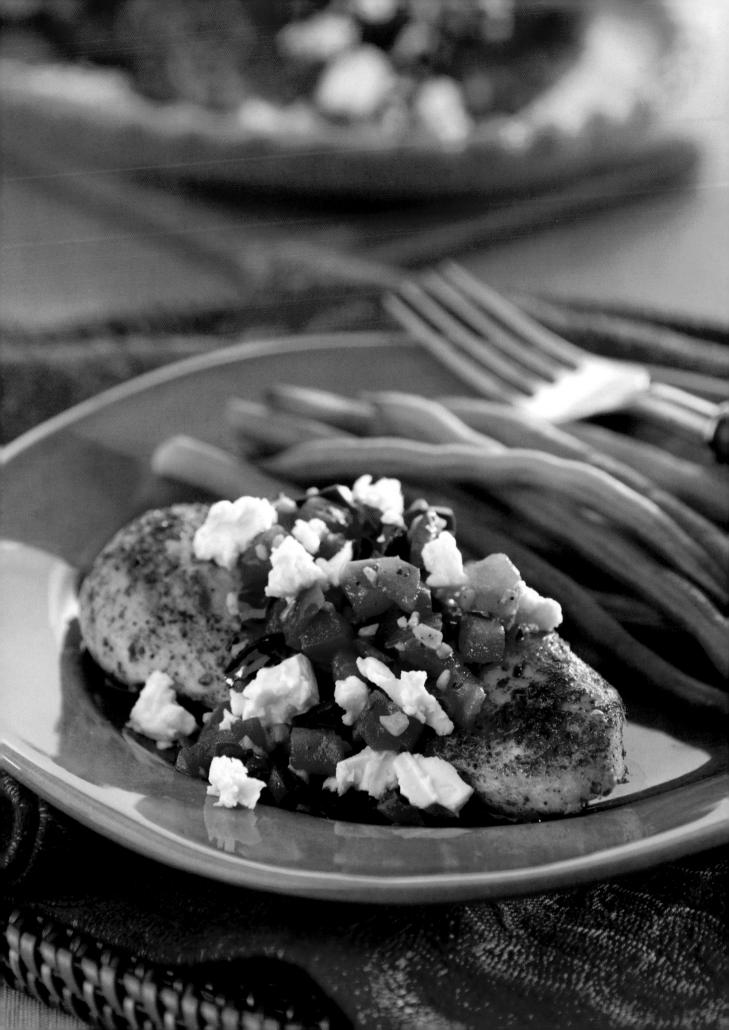

CHICKEN BREASTS WITH TOMATO-KALAMATA SAUCE

SERVES 4; 3 ounces chicken and 2 tablespoons sauce per serving

- 1 teaspoon dried oregano, crumbled
- ½ teaspoon paprika
- ½ teaspoon chili powder
- 4 boneless, skinless chicken breast halves (about 4 ounces each), all visible fat discarded
- 1 teaspoon olive or canola oil
- ½ cup water
- 1 medium tomato, seeded if desired and chopped
- 12 kalamata olives, coarsely chopped
- 1 medium garlic clove, minced
- ¼ teaspoon pepper
- ⅛ teaspoon salt
- 1½ ounces reduced-fat feta cheese, crumbled

In a small bowl, stir together the oregano, paprika, and chili powder. Sprinkle over the chicken. Using your fingertips, press the mixture firmly onto the chicken so the mixture adheres.

In a large nonstick skillet, heat the oil over medium heat, swirling to coat the bottom. Cook the chicken with the smooth side down for 5 minutes. Turn and cook for 4 minutes, or until the chicken is no longer pink in the center. Transfer to a serving plate.

Put the remaining ingredients except the feta in the skillet. Stir. Increase the heat to medium high and bring to a boil, scraping the bottom and side of the skillet to dislodge any browned bits. Boil for 2½ to 3 minutes, or until the sauce is reduced to ½ cup, stirring frequently. Spoon over the chicken. Sprinkle with the feta.

Nutrients per Serving: Calories 196, Total Fat 7.0 g, Saturated Fat 1.5 g, Polyunsaturated Fat 1.0 g, Monounsaturated Fat 3.5 g, Cholesterol 70 mg, Sodium 476 mg, Carbohydrates 4 g, Fiber 1 g, Sugars 1 g, Protein 29 g

Dietary Exchanges: 1 vegetable, 3½ lean meat

CAJUN CHICKEN AND RICE

SERVES 4; 3 ounces chicken and 1 cup rice mixture per serving

Vegetable oil spray
1 teaspoon olive oil
4 boneless, skinless chicken breast halves (about 4 ounces each), all visible fat discarded
1 teaspoon olive oil
1 medium red bell pepper, finely chopped
1 medium green bell pepper, finely chopped
¾ cup thinly sliced celery
½ medium onion, chopped
1 cup fat-free, low-sodium chicken broth
½ cup uncooked instant brown rice
¾ teaspoon Cajun seasoning blend
½ teaspoon dried thyme, crumbled
½ teaspoon Cajun seasoning blend
1 tablespoon olive oil (extra-virgin preferred)
¼ teaspoon salt

Preheat the oven to 350°F. Lightly spray an 11×7×2-inch glass baking dish with vegetable oil spray.

Heat 1 teaspoon oil in a large nonstick skillet over medium-high heat, swirling to coat the bottom. Cook the chicken on one side for 2 minutes, or until lightly browned. Transfer to a plate and set aside.

Pour 1 teaspoon oil into the skillet, swirling to coat the bottom. Cook the bell peppers, celery, and onion for 4 minutes, or until the onion is soft, stirring frequently. Stir in the broth, rice, ¾ teaspoon seasoning blend, and thyme. Increase the heat to high and bring to a boil. Transfer to the baking dish, spreading to cover the bottom.

Place the chicken pieces with the browned side up on the rice mixture. Sprinkle with ½ teaspoon seasoning blend. Cover with aluminum foil and bake for 30 minutes, or until the liquid is absorbed. Remove from the oven.

Transfer the chicken to the center of a serving platter. Stir the remaining oil and salt into the rice mixture. Spoon around the chicken.

Nutrients per Serving: Calories 246, Total Fat 7.5 g, Saturated Fat 1.0 g, Polyunsaturated Fat 1.0 g, Monounsaturated Fat 4.5 g, Cholesterol 66 mg, Sodium 405 mg, Carbohydrates 15 g, Fiber 3 g, Sugars 3 g, Protein 29 g

Dietary Exchanges: ½ starch, 1½ vegetable, 3 lean meat

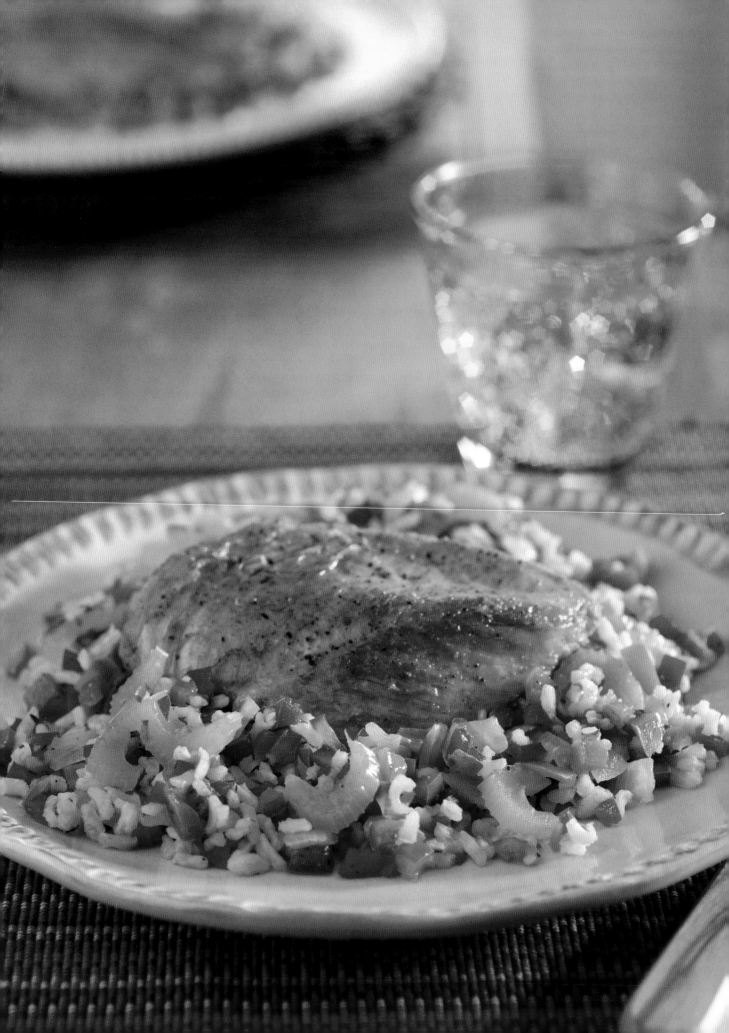

LIGHT AND EASY
CHICKEN STROGANOFF

SERVES 4; 1½ cups per serving

- 5 ounces dried no-yolk egg noodles
- 2 teaspoons dried dillweed, crumbled
  Vegetable oil spray
- 6 ounces sliced button mushrooms
- 2 cups diced cooked skinless chicken breasts, cooked without salt
- 1 10.75-ounce can low-fat, reduced-sodium condensed cream of chicken soup
- 2 medium green onions, finely chopped (green and white parts)
- 1 teaspoon Dijon mustard
- ¼ cup fat-free or low-fat plain yogurt or fat-free or light sour cream

Prepare the noodles using the package directions, omitting the salt and oil and adding the dillweed. Drain well.

Meanwhile, heat a 12-inch nonstick skillet over medium heat. Remove from the heat and lightly spray with vegetable oil spray (being careful not to spray near a gas flame). Cook the mushrooms for 5 minutes, or until limp, stirring frequently.

Stir in the chicken, soup, green onions, and mustard. Cook for 2 minutes, or until thoroughly heated.

Stir the noodles into the chicken mixture. Stir in the yogurt.

Nutrients per Serving: Calories 323, Total Fat 4.5 g, Saturated Fat 1.5 g, Polyunsaturated Fat 0.5 g, Monounsaturated Fat 1.0 g, Cholesterol 66 mg, Sodium 407 mg, Carbohydrates 38 g, Fiber 3 g, Sugars 5 g, Protein 30 g

Dietary Exchanges: 2½ starch, ½ fat

HOISIN CHICKEN CUTLETS

SERVES 4; 3 ounces chicken per serving

Sauce

  2 tablespoons hoisin sauce
  1 tablespoon no-salt-added ketchup
  1 tablespoon fresh orange juice
  1 tablespoon honey
  1 large garlic clove, minced

• • •

  2 tablespoons all-purpose flour
  1 tablespoon snipped fresh parsley
  ½ teaspoon garlic powder
  ⅛ to ¼ teaspoon cayenne
  4 boneless, skinless chicken breast halves or turkey cutlets (about 4 ounces each), all visible fat discarded
  1 tablespoon olive oil
  1 to 2 tablespoons sesame seeds, dry-roasted

In a small bowl, stir together the sauce ingredients. Set aside.

In a shallow bowl, stir together the flour, parsley, garlic powder, and cayenne.

Put a chicken breast half with the smooth side up between two pieces of wax paper or plastic wrap. Using a tortilla press, the smooth side of a meat mallet, or a rolling pin, lightly flatten the breasts to a thickness of ¼ inch, being careful not to tear the meat. (No flattening is needed for the turkey cutlets.) Coat with the flour mixture, shaking off the excess.

Heat a large nonstick skillet over medium-high heat. Pour the oil into the skillet and swirl to coat the bottom. Cook the chicken for 4 minutes. Turn the chicken. Spoon the hoisin sauce mixture over the chicken, spreading to cover. (Some of the sauce will run off into the pan.) Cook for 4 minutes, or until the chicken is no longer pink in the center. Sprinkle with the sesame seeds.

Nutrients per Serving: Calories 224, Total Fat 7.0 g, Saturated Fat 1.0 g, Polyunsaturated Fat 1.5 g, Monounsaturated Fat 3.5 g, Cholesterol 66 mg, Sodium 117 mg, Carbohydrates 12 g, Fiber 1 g, Sugars 8 g, Protein 28 g

Dietary Exchanges: 1 other carbohydrate, 3 lean meat

ROSEMARY-DIJON CHICKEN

SERVES 4; 1 chicken breast half per serving

- 2 tablespoons Dijon mustard (coarse ground preferred)
- 2 teaspoons olive oil
- ½ teaspoon dried rosemary, crushed, or dried tarragon, crumbled
- ¼ teaspoon salt
- ¼ teaspoon red hot-pepper sauce
  Vegetable oil spray
- 4 skinless chicken breast halves with bone (about 6 ounces each), all visible fat discarded

Preheat the oven to 350°F.

In a small bowl, stir together the mustard, oil, rosemary, salt, and hot-pepper sauce.

Spray a 13×9×2-inch baking pan with vegetable oil spray. Place the chicken in a single layer in the dish. Spoon the mustard mixture over each breast.

Bake for 40 to 45 minutes, or until the chicken is no longer pink in the center. Place the chicken on plates.

To serve, stir the pan drippings to dislodge any browned bits. Pour over the chicken.

Nutrients per Serving:
Calories 180, Total Fat 4.5 g,
Saturated Fat 1.0 g, Polyunsaturated
Fat 0.5 g, Monounsaturated
Fat 2.0 g, Cholesterol 79 mg,
Sodium 389 mg, Carbohydrates 1 g,
Fiber 0 g, Sugars 1 g, Protein 32 g

Dietary Exchanges:
4 very lean meat

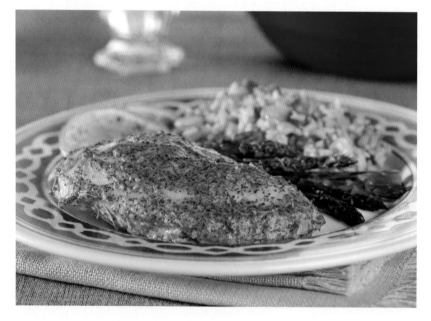

ROASTED TURKEY BREAST WITH LIME AND HERBS

SERVES 8; 3 ounces turkey per serving

        Vegetable oil spray
1   3½-pound turkey breast half with skin, thawed if frozen
3   tablespoons fresh lime juice
2   tablespoons olive oil
4   medium garlic cloves, minced
1   teaspoon dried oregano, crumbled
½   teaspoon dried tarragon, crumbled
½   teaspoon salt
½   teaspoon red hot-pepper sauce
¼   teaspoon pepper
¼   cup finely snipped fresh parsley

Lightly spray a large glass baking dish with vegetable oil spray. Put the turkey in the baking dish.

In a small bowl, stir together the remaining ingredients except the parsley. Stir in the parsley.

Using a tablespoon or your fingers, gently loosen the skin from the breast meat, creating a pocket. Being careful to not break the skin, spoon the parsley mixture as evenly as possible under the skin. Gently pull the skin over any exposed meat. Cover tightly with plastic wrap and refrigerate for 8 to 12 hours.

Preheat the oven to 325°F. Remove the plastic wrap from the turkey.

Roast the turkey with the skin side up for 1 hour 30 minutes to 1 hour 45 minutes, or until a meat thermometer or instant-read thermometer inserted into the thickest part of the breast registers 170°F and the juices run clear. Transfer to a cutting board. Let stand for 15 minutes for easier slicing and to let the turkey continue cooking (the internal temperature will rise at least 5°F). Discard the skin before eating the turkey.

Nutrients per Serving: Calories 187, Total Fat 4.5 g, Saturated Fat 1.0 g, Polyunsaturated Fat 0.5 g, Monounsaturated Fat 2.5 g, Cholesterol 93 mg, Sodium 209 mg, Carbohydrates 1 g, Fiber 0 g, Sugars 0 g, Protein 33 g
Dietary Exchanges: 4½ very lean meat

Meats

TEX-MEX BEEF, CORN, AND BROWN RICE

SERVES 4; 1½ cups per serving

1 teaspoon olive or canola oil
1 large onion, chopped
1 pound extra-lean ground beef
1 cup water
½ cup uncooked instant brown rice
1 10-ounce package frozen whole-kernel corn (2 cups)
1 medium tomato, chopped
½ to 1 chipotle pepper canned in adobo sauce, minced
½ 1- to 1.25-ounce packet taco seasoning mix (lowest sodium available)
2 tablespoons snipped cilantro
⅛ teaspoon salt
Snipped cilantro or cilantro leaves for garnish

In a large nonstick skillet, heat the oil over medium-high heat, swirling to coat the bottom. Cook the onion for 1 minute, stirring frequently. Add the beef. Cook for about 5 minutes, or until browned, breaking it up with a spoon and stirring constantly. Pour into a colander and drain if needed.

Stir in the water, rice, corn, tomato, and chipotle. Increase the heat to high and bring to a boil. Reduce the heat and simmer, covered, for 5 minutes, or until the rice is soft and most of the liquid is absorbed. Remove from the heat.

Stir in the taco seasoning, 2 tablespoons cilantro, and salt. Let stand, covered, for 5 minutes so the liquid and flavors are absorbed. Spoon onto plates. Sprinkle with the remaining cilantro.

Nutrients per Serving: Calories 313, Total Fat 8.0 g, Saturated Fat 2.5 g, Polyunsaturated Fat 1.0 g, Monounsaturated Fat 3.5 g, Cholesterol 62 mg, Sodium 458 mg, Carbohydrates 34 g, Fiber 4 g, Sugars 7 g, Protein 29 g

Dietary Exchanges: 2 starch, 1 vegetable, 3 lean meat

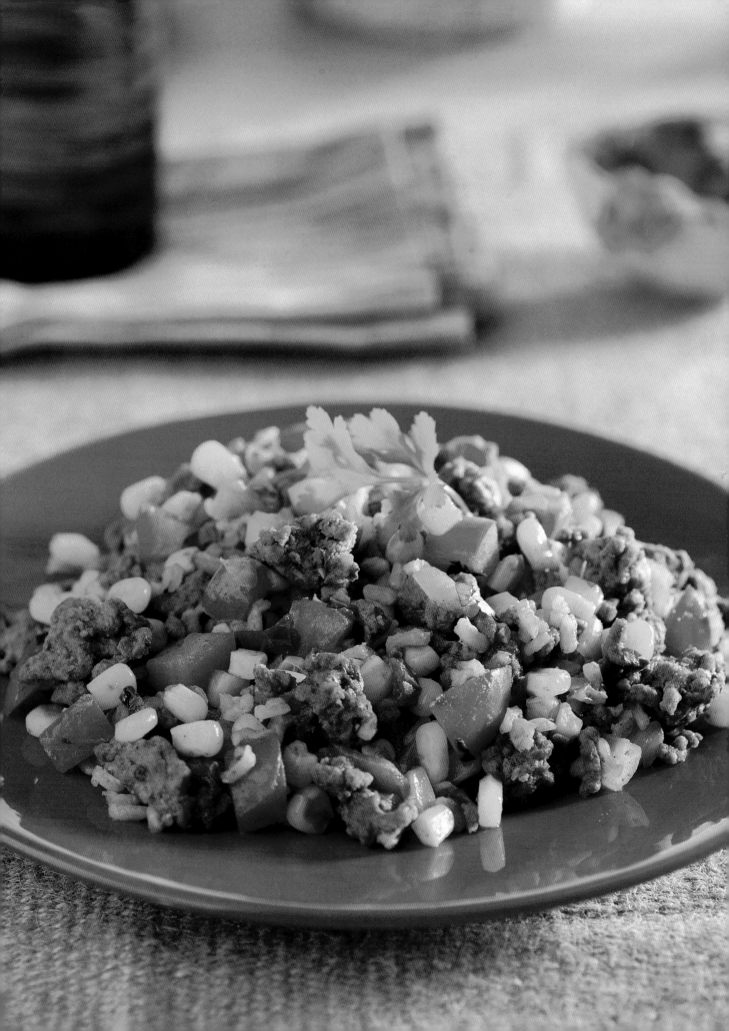

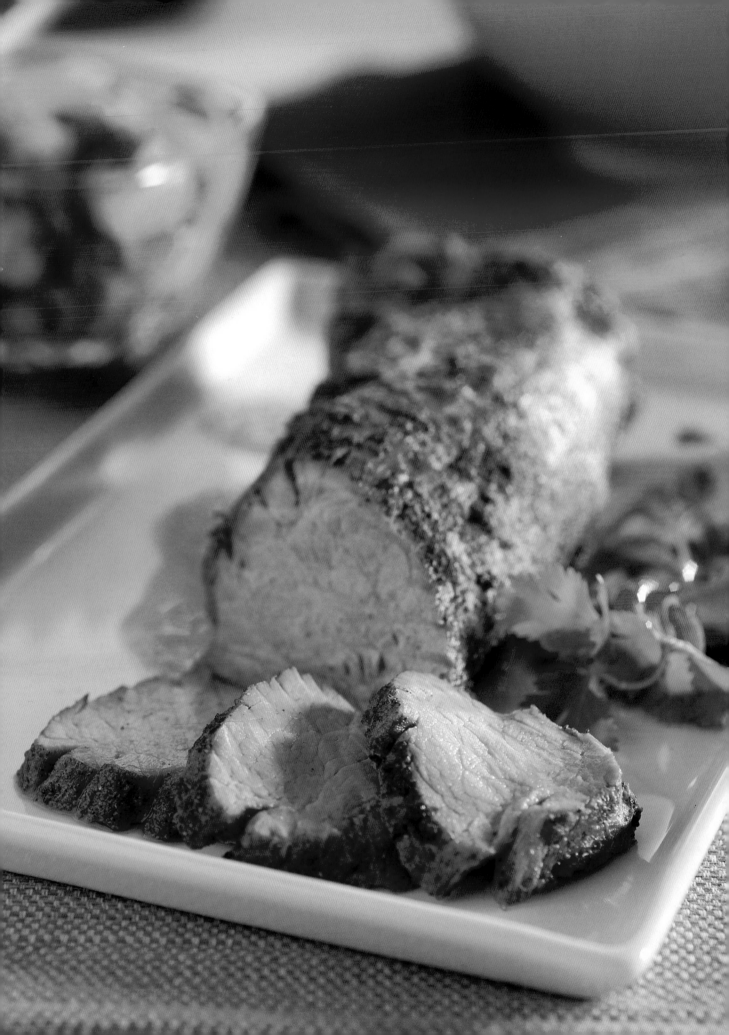

PORK TENDERLOIN WITH WARM FRUIT SALSA

SERVES 4; 3 ounces pork and ½ cup salsa per serving

- 1 teaspoon curry powder
- ½ teaspoon ground cumin
- ¼ teaspoon ground allspice
- ¼ teaspoon salt
- 1 1-pound pork tenderloin
- 2 teaspoons olive or canola oil, divided use
- ½ medium red bell pepper, finely chopped
- ¼ cup finely chopped red onion
- 1 medium jalapeño, seeded and finely chopped
- 1 8-ounce can pineapple tidbits in their own juice, well drained
- ¼ cup golden raisins
- 2 tablespoons snipped cilantro (optional)

In a small bowl, stir together the curry powder, cumin, allspice, and salt. Sprinkle the mixture all over the pork and press down lightly so the seasonings adhere. Let stand for 15 minutes.

Meanwhile, preheat the oven to 425°F.

In a large nonstick skillet, heat 1 teaspoon oil over medium-high heat, swirling to coat the bottom. Brown the pork for about 1 minute on each side, 4 to 5 minutes total. Transfer to an 11×7×2-inch glass baking dish. Bake for about 15 minutes, or until barely pink in the center. Place on a cutting board and let stand for 5 minutes, for easier slicing. Slice the pork, being sure to save the juice.

While the pork stands, wipe the skillet with a damp paper towel. Pour in the remaining 1 teaspoon oil and heat over medium-high heat, swirling to coat the bottom. Cook the bell pepper, onion, and jalapeño for 2 to 3 minutes, or until tender-crisp, stirring frequently. Stir in the pineapple, raisins, and cilantro. Cook for 1 minute, or until thoroughly heated. Remove from the heat.

To serve, transfer the pork slices to plates. Drizzle with the reserved juice. Serve the fruit salsa on the side.

Nutrients per Serving: Calories 203, Total Fat 5.0 g, Saturated Fat 1.5 g, Polyunsaturated Fat 0.5 g, Monounsaturated Fat 2.5 g, Cholesterol 63 mg, Sodium 197 mg, Carbohydrates 17 g, Fiber 2 g, Sugars 12 g, Protein 23 g

Dietary Exchanges: 1 fruit, 3 lean meat

MEAT LOAF

SERVES 6; 1 slice meat loaf and ¼ cup topping per serving

Vegetable oil spray

Meat Loaf

Whites of 2 large eggs

1 pound lean ground beef

½ cup uncooked oatmeal (regular preferred)

½ medium carrot, grated

1 small onion, chopped

2 tablespoons fat-free milk

1 tablespoon snipped fresh parsley (Italian [flat-leaf] preferred)

2 teaspoons Worcestershire sauce (lowest sodium available)

1 teaspoon olive oil

1 large garlic clove, minced

¼ teaspoon salt

¼ teaspoon pepper

Glaze

¼ cup no-salt-added ketchup

1 tablespoon firmly packed light brown sugar

1 tablespoon bottled chili sauce (lowest sodium available)

Tomato Topping

3 medium Italian plum tomatoes, chopped

2 tablespoons snipped fresh cilantro

1 tablespoon snipped fresh parsley (Italian [flat-leaf] preferred)

1 teaspoon olive oil

Preheat the oven to 350°F. Lightly spray a broiler pan and rack with vegetable oil spray.

In a large bowl, lightly beat the egg whites with a fork. Add the remaining meat loaf ingredients. Using your hands or a potato masher, combine thoroughly. Put the mixture on the broiler pan. Shape into an 8×3½×2-inch loaf.

In a small bowl, stir together the glaze ingredients. Spoon over the meat loaf. Bake for 1 hour 10 minutes, or until the meat loaf reaches an internal temperature of 160°F on an instant-read thermometer. Let stand for 5 minutes before slicing.

Meanwhile, in a small bowl, stir together the tomato topping ingredients. Spoon over the meat loaf.

Nutrients per Serving: Calories 220, Total Fat 10.0 g, Saturated Fat 3.0 g, Polyunsaturated Fat 0.5 g, Monounsaturated Fat 4.0 g, Cholesterol 43 mg, Sodium 186 mg, Carbohydrates 15 g, Fiber 2 g, Sugars 8 g, Protein 18 g

Dietary Exchanges: 1 starch, 2½ lean meat

SIRLOIN WITH PINEAPPLE-SHERRY MARINADE

SERVES 4; 3 ounces steak per serving

Marinade

¼ cup pineapple juice

¼ cup dry sherry

2 tablespoons firmly packed dark brown sugar

3 tablespoons light soy sauce

½ teaspoon chili garlic sauce or ⅛ to ¼ teaspoon crushed red pepper flakes

½ teaspoon ground cinnamon

¼ teaspoon ground allspice

• • •

1 1-pound boneless top sirloin steak, all visible fat discarded
Vegetable oil spray

¼ teaspoon pepper (coarsely ground preferred)

⅛ teaspoon salt

In a large resealable plastic bag, combine the marinade ingredients, making sure the sugar is dissolved. Add the sirloin. Seal the bag and turn to coat. Refrigerate for 8 to 24 hours, turning occasionally.

Preheat the broiler. Lightly spray a broiler rack and pan with vegetable oil spray. Remove the steak from the marinade, discarding the marinade. Place the steak on the broiler rack and broil at least 6 inches from the heat for 5 minutes on each side, or until the desired doneness. Transfer the steak to a cutting board. Sprinkle with the pepper and salt. Let stand for 5 minutes before slicing.

Nutrients per Serving: Calories 154, Total Fat 4.5 g, Saturated Fat 1.5 g, Polyunsaturated Fat 0.0 g, Monounsaturated Fat 2.0 g, Cholesterol 46 mg, Sodium 436 mg, Carbohydrates 1 g, Fiber 0 g, Sugars 0 g, Protein 25 g

Dietary Exchanges: 3 lean meat

Cook's Tip

Chili garlic sauce is a tangy, spicy blend of vinegar, spices, sugar, and, of course, chiles and garlic. Look for bottles of this slightly hot sauce in the Asian section of your supermarket.

SLOW-COOKER BEEF AND VEGGIES

SERVES 4; 1 cup beef mixture and ½ cup noodles per serving

Vegetable oil spray
1 pound boneless round steak (top or bottom), all visible fat discarded, cut into 1-inch cubes
¼ cup dry red wine (regular or nonalcoholic)
1½ cups baby carrots
1 medium onion, cut into 8 wedges
1 medium green bell pepper, cut into 1-inch pieces
1 tablespoon chili powder
1 teaspoon dried oregano, crumbled
¾ cup water
1 4-ounce can no-salt-added tomato sauce
1 0.87-ounce packet onion gravy mix
¼ teaspoon salt
4 ounces dried no-yolk egg noodles
¼ cup finely snipped fresh parsley

Lightly spray a slow cooker with vegetable oil spray.

Heat a large nonstick skillet over high heat. Remove from the heat and lightly spray with vegetable oil spray (being careful not to spray near a gas flame). Cook the beef for 3 minutes, or until beginning to brown, stirring constantly. Put the beef in the slow cooker.

Add the wine to the skillet. Cook over high heat for 30 seconds, scraping to dislodge any browned bits from the bottom. Pour over the beef.

Add the carrots, onion, bell pepper, chili powder, and oregano. Cook, covered, on high for 3 hours.

In a medium bowl, stir together the water, tomato sauce, gravy mix, and salt. Stir into the beef mixture. Cook, covered, for 30 minutes.

Meanwhile, prepare the noodles using the package directions, omitting the salt and oil. Drain well.

To serve, spoon the noodles onto plates or into shallow bowls. Spoon the beef mixture over the noodles. Sprinkle with the parsley.

Nutrients per Serving: Calories 337, Total Fat 4.5 g, Saturated Fat 1.5 g, Polyunsaturated Fat 0.5 g, Monounsaturated Fat 1.5 g, Cholesterol 64 mg, Sodium 497 mg, Carbohydrates 39 g, Fiber 5 g, Sugars 8 g, Protein 32 g

Dietary Exchanges: 1½ starch, 2½ vegetable, 3 very lean meat

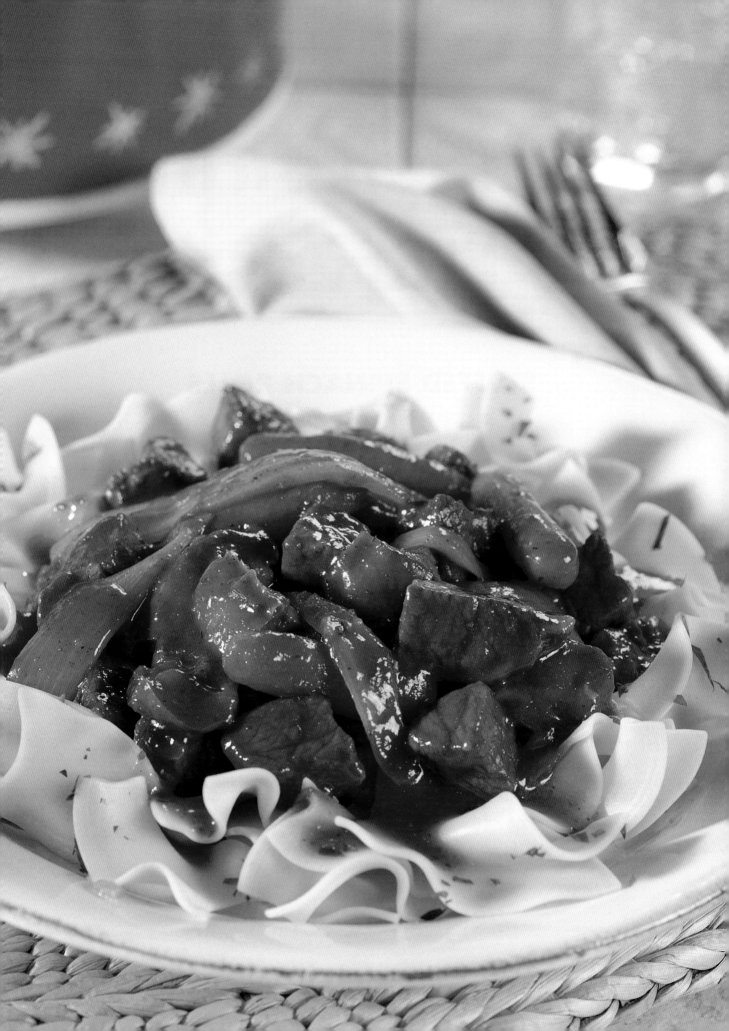

Vegetarian Entrées

STUFFED SPINACH ROLLS

SERVES 4; 1 roll per serving

Vegetable oil spray
- 4 dried whole-wheat lasagna noodles
- 10 ounces frozen chopped spinach, thawed and squeezed dry
- 1 cup fat-free or low-fat cottage cheese
- 1 tablespoon dried basil, crumbled
- ⅛ teaspoon salt
- ⅛ teaspoon crushed red pepper flakes
- 1 cup fat-free, low-sodium spaghetti sauce
- ½ cup shredded fat-free or part-skim mozzarella cheese
- 2 tablespoons shredded or grated Parmesan cheese

Preheat the oven to 350°F. Lightly spray an 11×7×2-inch baking dish with vegetable oil spray.

Prepare the noodles using the package directions, omitting the salt and oil. Drain well. Blot excess water with paper towels.

Meanwhile, in a medium bowl, stir together the spinach, cottage cheese, basil, salt, and red pepper flakes.

To assemble, place the noodles on a flat surface. Spread the spinach mixture over each noodle. Starting at one short end, roll up each noodle. Place seam side down in the baking dish, leaving about ½ inch between rolls. Spoon the spaghetti sauce over all. Sprinkle with the mozzarella.

Bake for 25 minutes, or until thoroughly heated. Sprinkle with the Parmesan.

Nutrients per Serving: Calories 203, Total Fat 2.0 g, Saturated Fat 0.5 g, Polyunsaturated Fat 0.0 g, Monounsaturated Fat 0.0 g, Cholesterol 7 mg, Sodium 581 mg, Carbohydrates 27 g, Fiber 7 g, Sugars 5 g, Protein 19 g

Dietary Exchanges: 1½ starch, 1 vegetable, 2 very lean meat

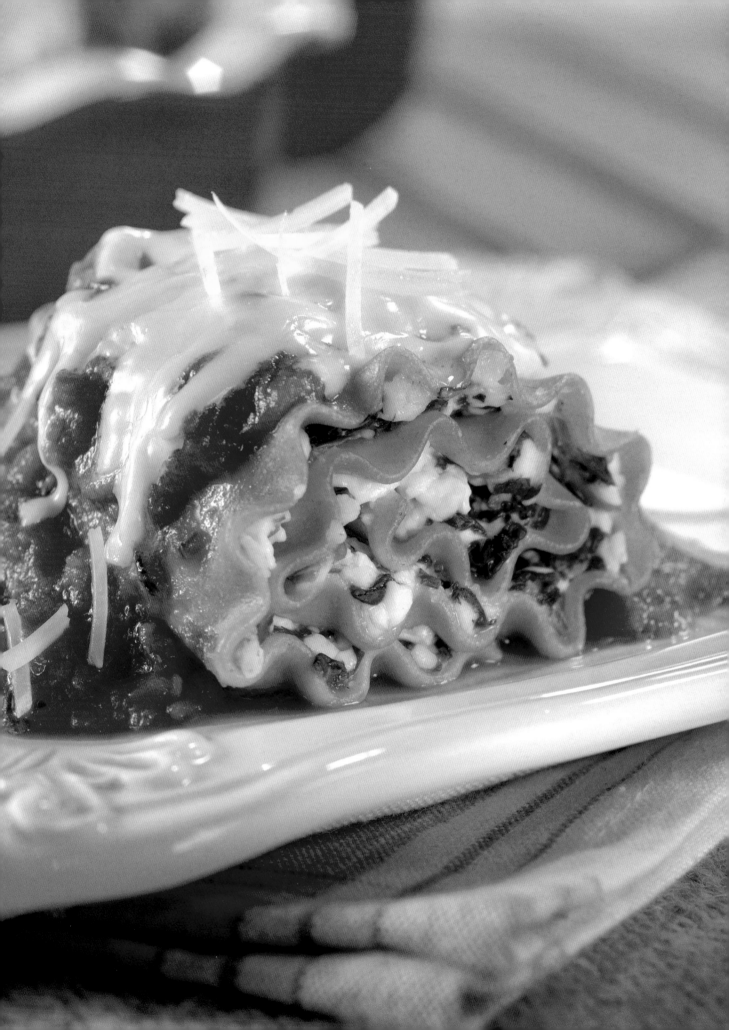

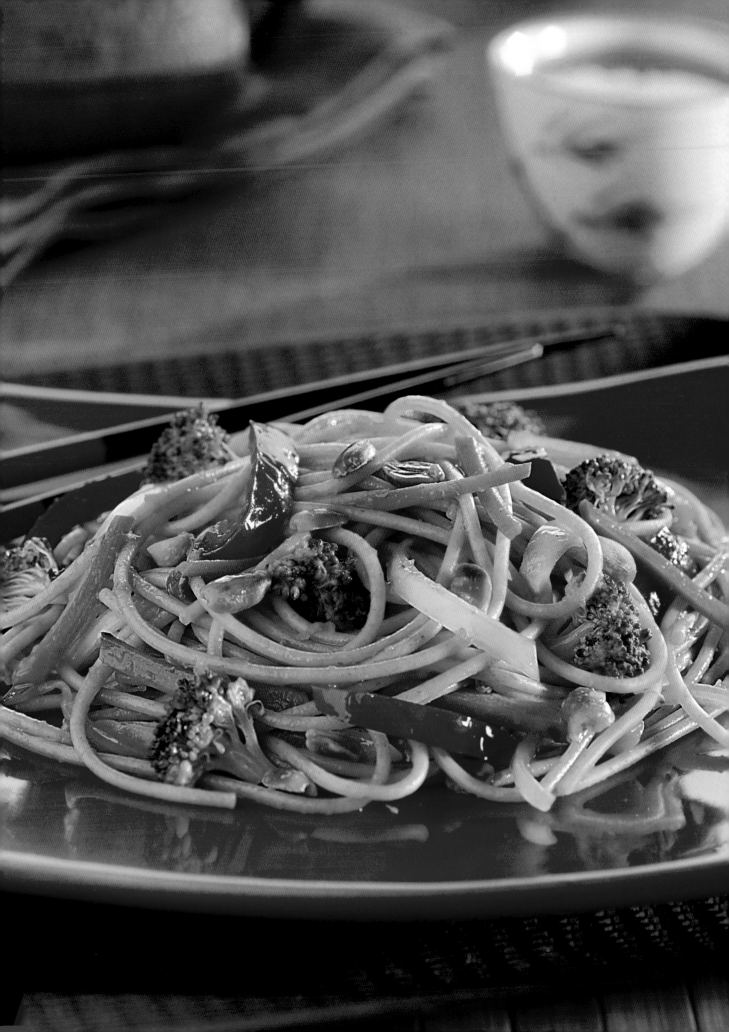

SWEET AND SPICY PEANUT-PASTA STIR-FRY

SERVES 4; 1½ cups per serving

- 5 ounces uncooked whole-wheat vermicelli or spaghetti, broken in half
- ½ teaspoon grated orange zest
- ⅓ cup fresh orange juice
- 3 tablespoons sugar
- 3 tablespoons light soy sauce
- 1 tablespoon cider vinegar
- 1 teaspoon grated peeled gingerroot
- ⅛ teaspoon crushed red pepper flakes (optional)
- ½ cup dry-roasted unsalted peanuts (about 2½ ounces)
- 1 teaspoon toasted sesame oil
- 2 cups small fresh broccoli florets (no larger than ¾ inch)
- 1 medium carrot, cut into matchstick-size pieces (about ¾ cup)
- 1 medium onion, cut into ¼-inch wedges
- 1 medium red bell pepper, cut into thin strips

Prepare the pasta using the package directions, omitting the salt and oil. Drain well.

Meanwhile, in a small bowl, stir together the orange zest, orange juice, sugar, soy sauce, vinegar, gingerroot, and red pepper flakes. Set aside.

Heat a large nonstick skillet over medium-high heat. Heat the peanuts for 2 minutes, or until they begin to lightly brown, stirring frequently. Transfer to a plate.

Add the oil to the same skillet and swirl to coat the bottom. Cook the broccoli, carrots, onion, and bell pepper for 6 minutes, or until just tender-crisp. Transfer to a large bowl. Stir in the cooked pasta and peanuts. Cover with aluminum foil to keep warm.

In the same skillet, bring the orange juice mixture to a boil. Cook for 2 minutes, or until reduced to about ⅓ cup, stirring constantly. Pour over the pasta mixture, stirring to blend.

Nutrients per Serving: Calories 331, Total Fat 10.5 g, Saturated Fat 1.5 g, Polyunsaturated Fat 3.5 g, Monounsaturated Fat 5.0 g, Cholesterol 0 mg, Sodium 321 mg, Carbohydrates 52 g, Fiber 9 g, Sugars 18 g, Protein 12 g

Dietary Exchanges: 2 starch, 2 vegetable, 1 other carbohydrate, ½ very lean meat, 1½ fat

THREE-CHEESE AND VEGETABLE CRUSTLESS QUICHE

SERVES 6; 1 wedge per serving

Vegetable oil spray

¾ cup shredded reduced-fat Cheddar cheese (about 3 ounces)

¾ cup shredded part-skim mozzarella cheese (about 3 ounces)

1 tablespoon olive oil, low-sodium vegetable broth, or fat-free, low-sodium chicken broth

½ cup thinly sliced button mushrooms

⅓ cup finely chopped onion

¾ cup frozen chopped spinach, thawed and squeezed dry

¾ cup frozen chopped broccoli or cauliflower, thawed and drained

Whites of 4 large eggs

½ cup egg substitute

¾ teaspoon salt-free all-purpose seasoning blend

10 drops red hot-pepper sauce

⅓ cup fat-free or low-fat cottage cheese

Preheat the oven to 375°F.

Lightly spray a 9-inch pie pan with vegetable oil spray. Put the Cheddar and mozzarella in the pie pan and stir together. Smooth the mixture over the bottom.

In a large nonstick skillet, heat the oil over medium-high heat, swirling to coat the bottom. Cook the mushrooms and onion for about 3 minutes, or until the onion is soft, stirring frequently. Reduce the heat to medium. Stir in the spinach and broccoli. Cook for 3 to 5 minutes, or until the vegetables are tender, stirring frequently. Pour into a colander and drain well if needed. Spoon over the cheeses and spread evenly.

In a medium bowl, whisk together the remaining ingredients except the cottage cheese until slightly frothy. Stir in the cottage cheese. Pour over the spinach mixture.

Bake for 30 to 35 minutes, or until the tip of a knife inserted in the center comes out clean. Remove from the oven and let stand for 5 minutes, or until set (doesn't jiggle when gently shaken), before slicing.

Nutrients per Serving: Calories 128, Total Fat 5.5 g, Saturated Fat 2.5 g, Polyunsaturated Fat 0.5 g, Monounsaturated Fat 2.5 g, Cholesterol 13 mg, Sodium 336 mg, Carbohydrates 5 g, Fiber 1 g, Sugars 3 g, Protein 15 g

Dietary Exchanges: 1 vegetable, 2 lean meat

MEDITERRANEAN WHITE BEANS AND BROWN RICE

SERVES 4; 1½ cups per serving

Vegetable oil spray
1½ cups chopped onions
1¾ cups water
1½ cups uncooked instant brown rice
1 cup grape tomatoes or cherry tomatoes
1 16-ounce can no-salt-added navy beans, rinsed and drained
½ cup snipped fresh parsley
1 tablespoon dried basil, crumbled
1 medium garlic clove, minced
¼ teaspoon salt
3 ounces fat-free or low-fat feta with sun-dried tomatoes and basil, crumbled

Heat a 12-inch nonstick skillet over medium-high heat. Remove from the heat and lightly spray with vegetable oil spray (being careful not to spray near a gas flame). Cook the onions for 4 minutes, or until soft, stirring frequently.

Add the water. Bring to a full boil over medium-high heat. Stir in the rice. Reduce the heat and simmer, covered, for 10 minutes, or until the water is absorbed. Remove from the heat.

Halve the grape tomatoes or quarter the cherry tomatoes. Stir the tomatoes and the remaining ingredients except the feta into the rice. Let stand, covered, for 5 minutes to heat thoroughly and absorb flavors. Gently stir in the feta.

Nutrients per Serving: Calories 287, Total Fat 1.5 g, Saturated Fat 0.0 g, Polyunsaturated Fat 0.5 g, Monounsaturated Fat 0.5 g, Cholesterol 0 mg, Sodium 502 mg, Carbohydrates 54 g, Fiber 8 g, Sugars 10 g, Protein 15 g

Dietary Exchanges: 3 starch, 1½ vegetable, 1 very lean meat

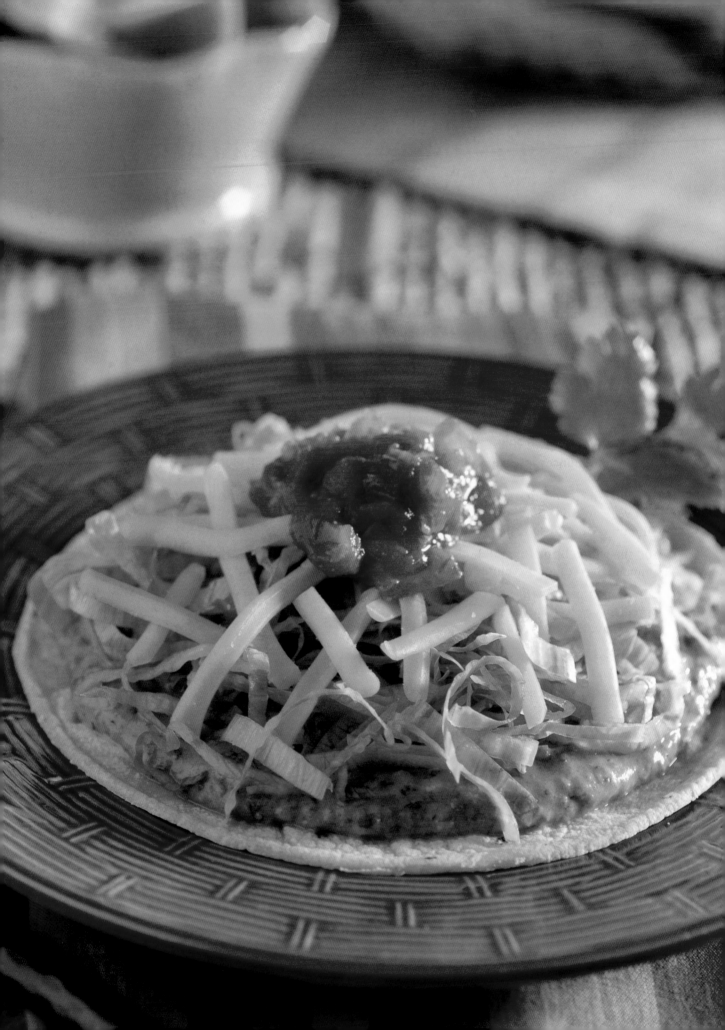

KNIFE-AND-FORK
BLACK BEAN TORTILLAS

SERVES 4; 1 tortilla per serving

1   15-ounce can no-salt-added black beans, rinsed and well drained
½   cup fat-free or light sour cream
¼   cup picante sauce (lowest sodium available)
1   teaspoon grated lime zest
3   tablespoons fresh lime juice
3   tablespoons coarsely chopped cilantro
2   tablespoons fat-free or light mayonnaise
1   medium garlic clove, minced
4   6-inch corn tortillas
2 to 3 cups shredded lettuce (about ½ 10-ounce package)
¾   cup shredded fat-free sharp Cheddar cheese (about 3 ounces)
¼   cup picante sauce (lowest sodium available)

In a food processor or blender, process the beans, sour cream, ¼ cup picante sauce, lime zest, lime juice, cilantro, mayonnaise, and garlic until smooth.

Using the directions on the package, warm the tortillas. Place a tortilla on each plate. Spoon about ½ cup bean mixture onto each tortilla. Spread the mixture. Top with the lettuce, Cheddar, and remaining picante sauce.

Nutrients per Serving: Calories 205, Total Fat 0.5 g, Saturated Fat 0.0 g, Polyunsaturated Fat 0.0 g, Monounsaturated Fat 0.0 g, Cholesterol 10 mg, Sodium 524 mg, Carbohydrates 34 g, Fiber 6 g, Sugars 7 g, Protein 16 g
Dietary Exchanges: 2½ starch, 2 very lean meat

Vegetables & Side Dishes

ASIAN GREEN BEANS

SERVES 4; ½ cup per serving

12 ounces fresh green beans, trimmed and cut diagonally into 2-inch pieces

½ cup thinly sliced red onion

1 tablespoon cider vinegar

2 teaspoons sugar

1 teaspoon grated peeled gingerroot

1 teaspoon toasted sesame oil

¼ teaspoon salt

⅛ teaspoon crushed red pepper flakes

In a large saucepan, steam the green beans and onion for 6 minutes, or until tender-crisp. Remove from the heat. Pour into a colander and drain well. Transfer to a serving bowl.

Add the remaining ingredients, stirring gently to coat.

Nutrients per Serving: Calories 51, Total Fat 1.0 g, Saturated Fat 0.0 g, Polyunsaturated Fat 0.5 g, Monounsaturated Fat 0.5 g, Cholesterol 0 mg, Sodium 146 mg, Carbohydrates 9 g, Fiber 3 g, Sugars 5 g, Protein 1 g

Dietary Exchanges: 2 vegetable

Cook's Tip

You can easily serve this dish as a salad. Let the green beans and onion cool, then toss them with the remaining ingredients, using double amounts of vinegar, sugar, and gingerroot.

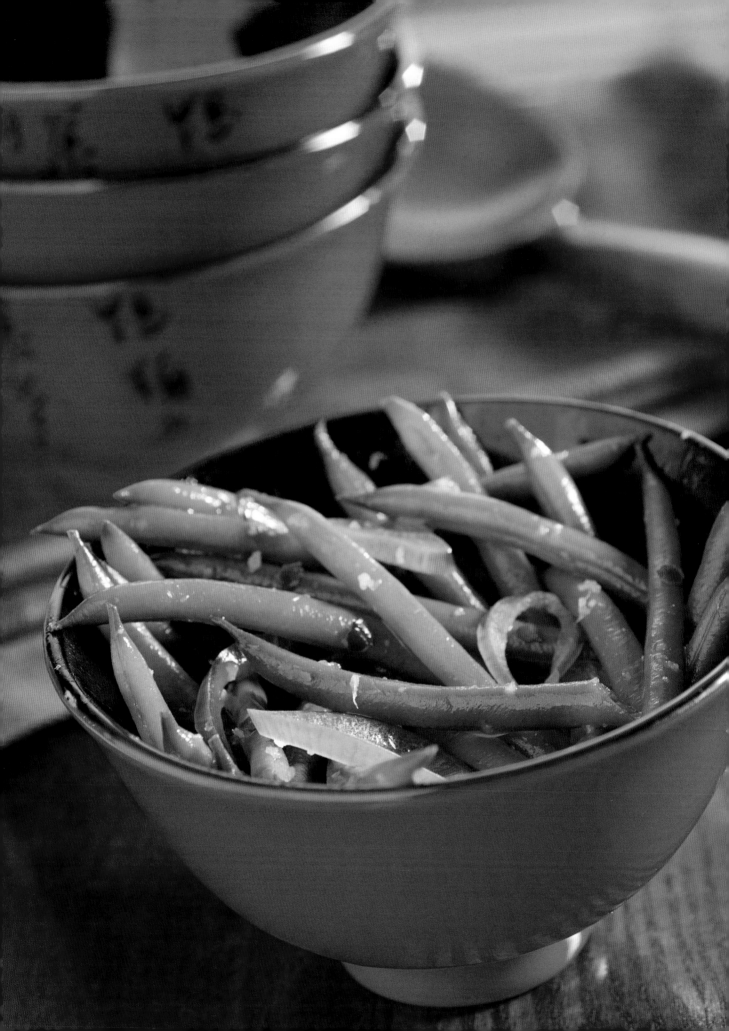

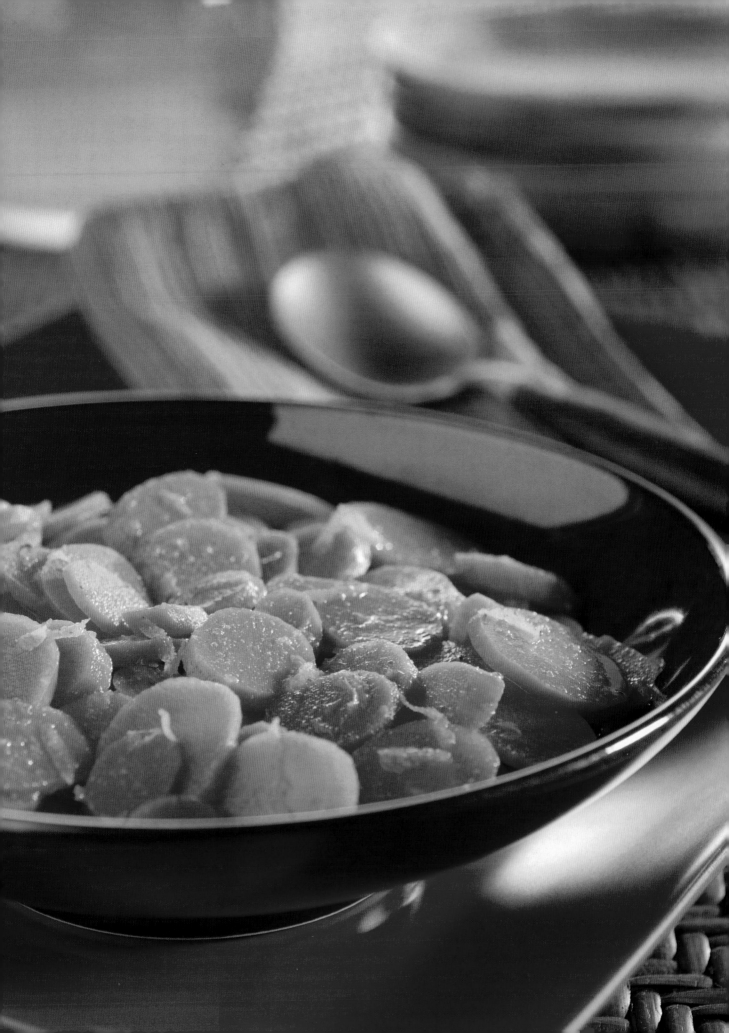

CARROTS WITH CURRY-FLAVORED ORANGE SAUCE

SERVES 4; ½ cup carrots and 1 tablespoon sauce per serving

4 medium carrots, cut diagonally into ⅛-inch slices

Sauce

⅓ cup fresh orange juice

½ teaspoon grated orange zest

2 tablespoons firmly packed dark brown sugar

1 tablespoon light tub margarine

½ teaspoon curry powder

⅛ teaspoon ground cumin

⅛ teaspoon salt

In a large saucepan, steam the carrots for 7 to 8 minutes, or until just tender. Pour into a colander and drain well. Transfer to a serving bowl.

Meanwhile, in a small saucepan, bring the orange juice to a boil over medium-high heat. Boil for 1½ minutes, or until reduced to 2 tablespoons. Remove from the heat. Stir in the remaining sauce ingredients. Pour over the carrots (no stirring needed).

Nutrients per Serving: Calories 76, Total Fat 1.5 g, Saturated Fat 0.0 g, Polyunsaturated Fat 0.5 g, Monounsaturated Fat 0.5 g, Cholesterol 0 mg, Sodium 148 mg, Carbohydrates 16 g, Fiber 2 g, Sugars 12 g, Protein 1 g
Dietary Exchanges: 1½ vegetable, ½ other carbohydrate

Cook's Tip

When you are boiling a liquid for a reduction, be sure to watch carefully. The bubbles created while the liquid is boiling can make it look like you have more sauce in the pan than you really do.

BROCCOLI WITH LEMON-WORCESTERSHIRE SAUCE

SERVES 4; ½ cup broccoli and scant 2 teaspoons sauce per serving

> 2 cups fresh broccoli florets or 10 ounces frozen broccoli spears
> ½ cup water (if using florets)

Sauce

> 2 tablespoons light tub margarine
> 1 teaspoon fresh lemon juice
> ½ teaspoon Worcestershire sauce (lowest sodium available)
> ⅛ teaspoon garlic powder
> ⅛ teaspoon salt

If using the florets, put them in a large skillet with the water. Bring to a boil over medium-high heat. Reduce the heat and simmer, covered, for 2 minutes. If using the spears, cook them using the package directions, omitting the salt and margarine, until fork tender. Using a slotted spoon or tongs, transfer the broccoli to paper towels. Drain well. Transfer to a serving plate.

Meanwhile, in a small skillet or saucepan, stir together the sauce ingredients. Heat over medium-low heat for about 30 seconds, or until the margarine has just melted. Stir to blend. Spoon over the broccoli (no stirring needed).

Nutrients per Serving: Calories 31, Total Fat 2.5 g, Saturated Fat 0.0 g, Polyunsaturated Fat 0.5 g, Monounsaturated Fat 1.5 g, Cholesterol 0 mg, Sodium 128 mg, Carbohydrates 2 g, Fiber 1 g, Sugars 0 g, Protein 1 g
Dietary Exchanges: ½ fat

ACORN SQUASH WITH APRICOTS AND RAISINS

SERVES 4; 1 squash wedge per serving

Vegetable oil spray

¼ cup water

1 1-pound acorn squash

¼ cup raisins

¼ cup chopped dried apricots

2 tablespoons firmly packed dark brown sugar

½ teaspoon ground cinnamon

½ teaspoon grated orange zest

¼ cup fresh orange juice

⅛ teaspoon salt

Spray a microwaveable 9-inch baking pan or deep-dish pie pan with vegetable oil spray. Pour the water into the pan.

Pierce the skin of the squash with a fork in several places so the squash won't dry out. Cut the squash in half vertically. Scoop out and discard the seeds and strings. Place the squash with the cut side up in the pan.

In a small bowl, stir together the remaining ingredients. Spoon onto each squash half. Cover the pan loosely with wax paper.

Microwave at 100 percent power (high) for 10 to 15 minutes, or until the squash is tender when pierced with a fork. Cut each squash half in half.

Nutrients per Serving: Calories 126, Total Fat 0.0 g, Saturated Fat 0.0 g, Polyunsaturated Fat 0.0 g, Monounsaturated Fat 0.0 g, Cholesterol 0 mg, Sodium 80 mg, Carbohydrates 32 g, Fiber 2 g, Sugars 20 g, Protein 2 g

Dietary Exchanges: 1 starch, 1 fruit

BROILED ASPARAGUS SPEARS WITH LEMON

SERVES 4; about 6 spears per serving

2 medium lemons, thinly sliced (about 8 slices each)
1 pound medium asparagus spears (about 24), trimmed
  Vegetable oil spray
2 teaspoons olive oil (extra-virgin preferred)
¼ teaspoon salt
⅛ teaspoon pepper

Preheat the broiler.

Line a broiler pan with aluminum foil. Arrange the lemon slices close together in a single layer in the pan. Arrange the asparagus spears in a single layer on the lemon slices. Lightly spray the asparagus with vegetable oil spray.

Broil about 4 inches from the heat source for 6 minutes, or until just tender-crisp.

Transfer the asparagus to a serving plate. Drizzle the oil over the asparagus. Sprinkle with the salt and pepper. Drizzle with any accumulated juices from the broiler pan. Place the lemon slices on or around the asparagus.

Nutrients per Serving: Calories 51, Total Fat 2.5 g, Saturated Fat 0.5 g, Polyunsaturated Fat 0.0 g, Monounsaturated Fat 1.5 g, Cholesterol 0 mg, Sodium 145 mg, Carbohydrates 5 g, Fiber 3 g, Sugars 2 g, Protein 2 g
Dietary Exchanges: 1 vegetable, ½ fat

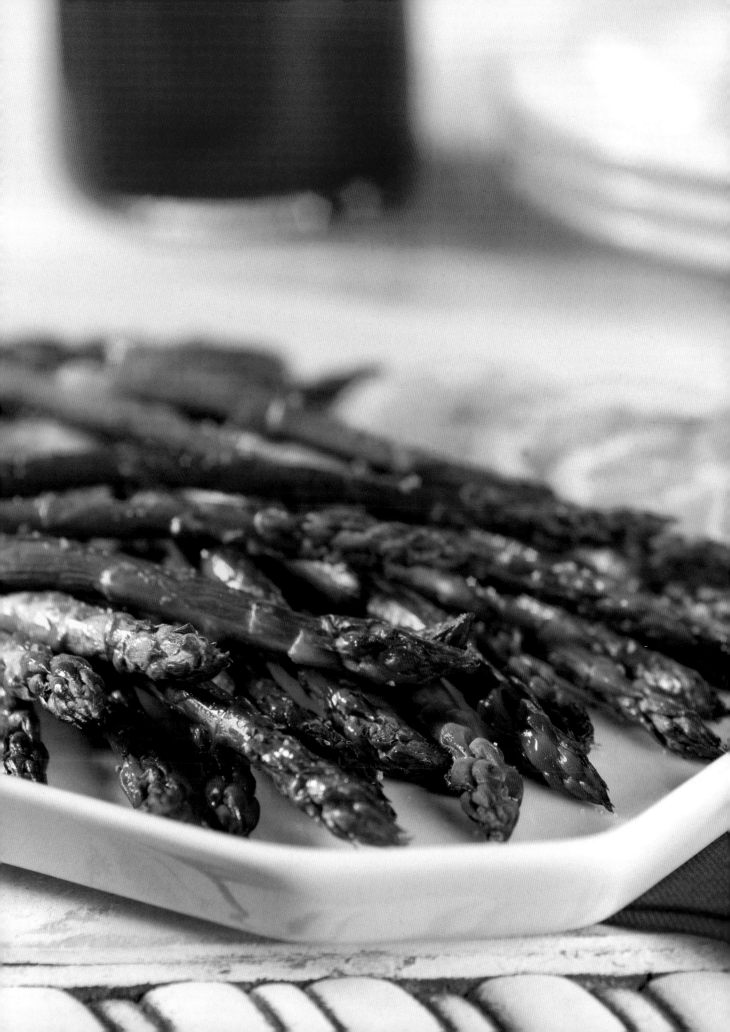

ROASTED SWEET POTATO CUBES

SERVES 4; about ⅔ cup per serving

Vegetable oil spray
1 pound sweet potatoes, peeled and cut into ¾-inch cubes
2 teaspoons canola or corn oil
2 tablespoons dark brown sugar
¼ teaspoon ground cinnamon
¼ teaspoon salt

Preheat the oven to 425°F.

Line a baking sheet with aluminum foil. Lightly spray the foil with vegetable oil spray. Put the sweet potatoes on the foil. Drizzle with the oil. Toss gently to coat. Arrange in a single layer.

Sprinkle with the remaining ingredients.

Bake for 15 minutes. Stir. Bake for 10 minutes, or until very tender when pierced with a fork.

Nutrients per Serving: Calories 133, Total Fat 2.5 g, Saturated Fat 0.0 g, Polyunsaturated Fat 1.0 g, Monounsaturated Fat 1.5 g, Cholesterol 0 mg, Sodium 159 mg, Carbohydrates 27 g, Fiber 3 g, Sugars 11 g, Protein 1 g
Dietary Exchanges: 2 starch

Cook's Tip

For the best texture, be sure to cook the potatoes for the full amount of time recommended.

BROWN RICE AND WALNUT PILAF

SERVES 4; ¾ cup per serving

1¼ cups fat-free, low-sodium chicken broth
1 cup uncooked quick-cooking brown rice
2 tablespoons walnut pieces
   Vegetable oil spray
1 large onion, chopped
½ medium red bell pepper, chopped
2 tablespoons snipped fresh cilantro
¼ teaspoon ground cumin
¼ teaspoon salt

In a small saucepan, bring the broth to a boil over high heat. Stir in the rice. Cook, covered, for the time called for in the package directions.

Meanwhile, heat a large nonstick skillet over medium-high heat. Dry-roast the walnuts for 2 to 3 minutes, or until just beginning to lightly brown, stirring constantly. Transfer to a small plate.

Lightly spray the skillet with vegetable oil spray. Cook the onion and bell pepper over medium-high heat for 6 minutes, or until richly brown, stirring frequently. Remove from the heat.

Stir in the remaining ingredients, including the rice and walnuts.

Nutrients per Serving: Calories 137, Total Fat 3.5 g, Saturated Fat 0.0 g, Polyunsaturated Fat 2.0 g, Monounsaturated Fat 0.5 g, Cholesterol 0 mg, Sodium 172 mg, Carbohydrates 23 g, Fiber 2 g, Sugars 3 g, Protein 4 g
Dietary Exchanges: 1 starch, 1½ vegetable, ½ fat

Breads & Breakfast Dishes

SPANISH OMELET

SERVES 4; 1 wedge per serving

1½ teaspoons olive oil

1½ teaspoons light tub margarine

1 medium onion, chopped

1 medium garlic clove, minced

4 cups frozen low-fat hash brown potatoes, thawed

½ medium red bell pepper, chopped

2 ounces chopped Canadian bacon (about ½ cup)

¾ cup egg substitute

1 large egg

⅛ teaspoon pepper

2 tablespoons snipped fresh parsley

In a medium nonstick skillet, heat the oil and margarine over medium-low heat until the margarine melts, swirling to coat the bottom. Cook the onion and garlic until the onion is soft, 4 to 5 minutes. Stir in the potatoes, bell pepper, and Canadian bacon. Cook for 1 minute.

Meanwhile, in a medium bowl, whisk together the egg substitute, egg, and pepper. Pour over the potato mixture, shaking the skillet to distribute the egg mixture evenly. Reduce the heat to low and cook, covered, for 10 to 13 minutes, or until the mixture is set but slightly liquid on top. If you don't wish to invert the omelet, cook it for an extra 2 to 3 minutes, covered, or until cooked through. Otherwise, invert the omelet onto a large plate, then slip it back into the skillet so the slightly liquid side is face down. Increase the heat to medium low and cook for 2 to 3 minutes, or until cooked through. Slip the omelet onto a platter. Sprinkle with the parsley before cutting.

Nutrients per Serving: Calories 266, Total Fat 4.5 g, Saturated Fat 1.0 g, Polyunsaturated Fat 0.5 g, Monounsaturated Fat 2.5 g, Cholesterol 60 mg, Sodium 371 mg, Carbohydrates 43 g, Fiber 4 g, Sugars 4 g, Protein 14 g

Dietary Exchanges: 2½ starch, 1 vegetable, 1½ very lean meat

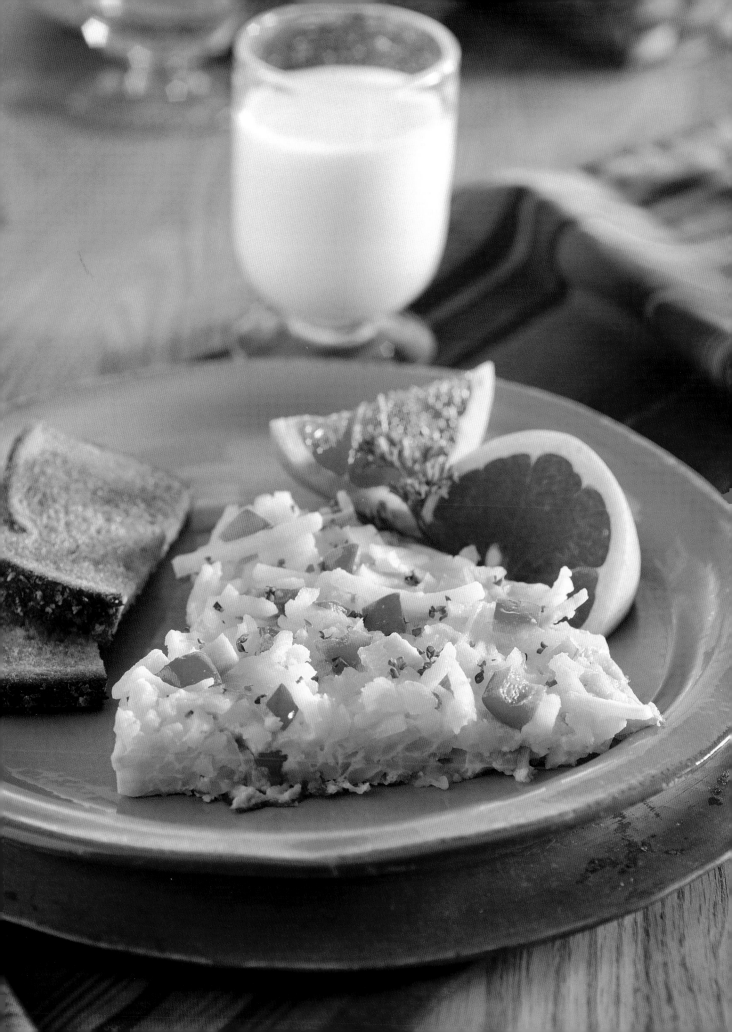

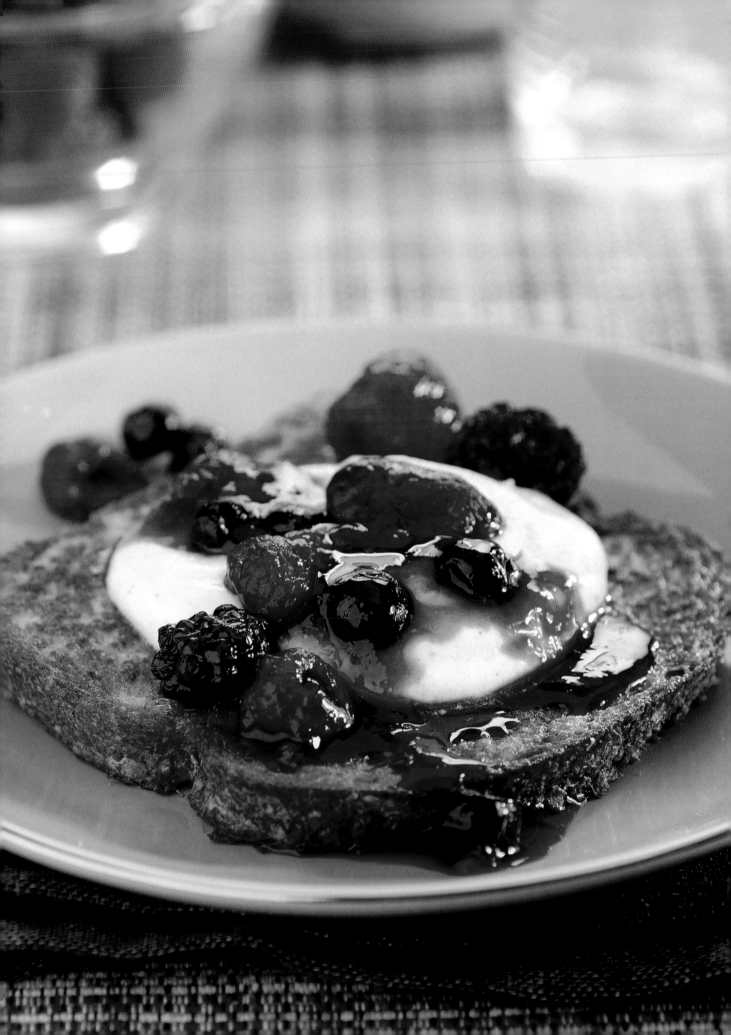

FRENCH TOAST WITH MIXED BERRIES

SERVES 4; 1 slice bread, ¼ cup topping, and ¼ cup berry mixture per serving

- 2 tablespoons seedless raspberry all-fruit spread
- 8 ounces frozen unsweetened mixed berries, thawed
- ¼ teaspoon vanilla extract
- ¾ cup egg substitute
- 3 tablespoons fat-free milk
- 1 teaspoon vanilla extract
- ½ teaspoon ground cinnamon
- 4 slices reduced-calorie whole-wheat bread
- 1 teaspoon canola or corn oil
- ⅔ cup fat-free or light frozen whipped topping, thawed in refrigerator
- ⅓ cup fat-free or low-fat vanilla yogurt
- ⅛ teaspoon ground cinnamon

In a medium microwaveable bowl, microwave the raspberry spread on 50 percent power (medium) for 15 to 20 seconds, or until just melted. Whisk until smooth. Gently stir in the berries and ¼ teaspoon vanilla. Set aside.

In a shallow pan, such as a pie pan, whisk together the egg substitute, milk, 1 teaspoon vanilla, and ½ teaspoon cinnamon. Dip each bread slice in the mixture, turning to coat both sides. Let the excess mixture drip back into the pan. Put the bread in a single layer on a plate.

Pour the oil into a large nonstick griddle or skillet. Using a paper towel, spread the oil over the bottom. Heat over medium heat. Put the bread in a single layer on the griddle. Cook for 3 minutes on each side, or until golden.

Meanwhile, in a medium bowl, stir together the whipped topping, yogurt, and ⅛ teaspoon cinnamon.

To serve, place a bread slice on each plate. Spoon the whipped topping mixture onto the center of each slice. Spoon the berry mixture over each serving.

Nutrients per Serving: Calories 168, Total Fat 1.5 g, Saturated Fat 0.0 g, Polyunsaturated Fat 0.5 g, Monounsaturated Fat 0.5 g, Cholesterol 1 mg, Sodium 234 mg, Carbohydrates 30 g, Fiber 5 g, Sugars 16 g, Protein 8 g
Dietary Exchanges: 1 starch, 1 fruit, 1 very lean meat

WHOLE-WHEAT CRANBERRY MUFFINS

SERVES 12; 1 muffin per serving

Vegetable oil spray (optional)
¾ cup uncooked quick-cooking oatmeal
½ cup whole-wheat flour
½ cup all-purpose flour
½ cup firmly packed light brown sugar
½ cup sweetened dried cranberries
¼ cup toasted wheat germ
2 teaspoons baking powder
¼ teaspoon baking soda
¾ cup pineapple juice
Egg substitute equivalent to 1 egg, or 1 large egg
1 tablespoon canola or corn oil
2 tablespoons unsalted sunflower seeds

Preheat the oven to 400°F. Lightly spray a 12-cup muffin pan with vegetable oil spray or put paper muffin cups in the pan.

In a medium bowl, stir together the oatmeal, flours, brown sugar, cranberries, wheat germ, baking powder, and baking soda. Make a well in the center. Pour the pineapple juice, egg substitute, and oil into the well, stirring until just moistened. Do not overmix; the batter should be slightly lumpy. Spoon the batter evenly into muffin cups. Sprinkle with the sunflower seeds.

Bake for 11 to 12 minutes, or until a cake tester or wooden toothpick inserted in the center of a muffin comes out clean. These muffins don't need a cooling time before removing from the pan.

Nutrients per Serving: Calories 143, Total Fat 2.5 g, Saturated Fat 0.5 g, Polyunsaturated Fat 1.0 g, Monounsaturated Fat 1.0 g, Cholesterol 0 mg, Sodium 108 mg, Carbohydrates 28 g, Fiber 2 g, Sugars 15 g, Protein 3 g
Dietary Exchanges: 2 starch

RASPBERRY-MANGO BREAKFAST PARFAITS

SERVES 4; ¾ cup yogurt, ½ cup fruit, and 2 tablespoons sauce per serving

- 2 cups fresh or frozen unsweetened raspberries, thawed if frozen
- 1 mango, diced (about 1½ cups)
- 4 6-ounce containers fat-free, sugar-free or low-fat, sugar-free vanilla yogurt
- 2 tablespoons sugar
- ½ teaspoon ground cinnamon

In each of 4 parfait glasses or wine goblets, spoon 2 tablespoons raspberries, 2 tablespoons mango, and a heaping ⅓ cup yogurt. Repeat the layers, using all the remaining yogurt.

In a blender or food processor, process the remaining raspberries and mango with the sugar and cinnamon until smooth. Spoon the pureed mixture over each serving, about 2 tablespoons each.

Nutrients per Serving: Calories 181, Total Fat 0.5 g, Saturated Fat 0.0 g, Polyunsaturated Fat 0.5 g, Monounsaturated Fat 0.0 g, Cholesterol 4 mg, Sodium 99 mg, Carbohydrates 38 g, Fiber 5 g, Sugars 28 g, Protein 6 g

Dietary Exchanges: 1 skim milk, 1½ fruit

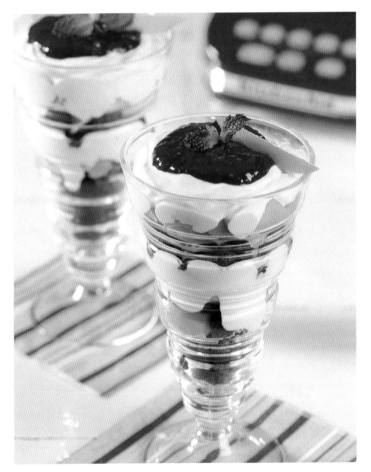

Desserts

CHERRY PHYLLO NESTS

SERVES 4; 2 phyllo nests, ¼ cup cherry filling, and 2 tablespoons ice cream per serving

    Vegetable oil spray (butter flavor preferred)
2 **sheets frozen phyllo dough, thawed**
1 **cup light cherry pie filling**
1 **teaspoon orange zest, divided**
½ **cup fat-free or light vanilla ice cream or frozen yogurt**

Preheat the oven to 350°F. Lightly spray a nonstick muffin pan with vegetable oil spray.

Lightly spray both sides of 1 sheet of phyllo with vegetable oil spray. (Follow the package directions about keeping the other sheet covered.) Working quickly, cut the dough into 4 lengthwise strips. Cut each strip crosswise into fourths to make 16 squares.

Place 4 squares in each of 4 muffin cups, with corners overlapping in the center. Press down gently on the bottom so the phyllo will mold to the shape of the cup. Ruffle the edges so the phyllo looks like a nest. Repeat with the remaining phyllo sheet, making 4 more nests.

Bake for 4 minutes, or until golden. Put the muffin pan on a cooling rack and let the nests cool completely. Gently remove the cooled nests from the muffin pan.

Combine the pie filling and ½ teaspoon orange zest. Fill each nest with 2 tablespoons pie filling. Using a melon baller, place 1 tablespoon-size ice cream ball on each nest. Garnish with the remaining ½ teaspoon orange zest. Serve immediately.

Nutrients per Serving: Calories 89, Total Fat 0.5 g, Saturated Fat 0.0 g, Polyunsaturated Fat 0.0 g, Monounsaturated Fat 0.0 g, Cholesterol 0 mg, Sodium 70 mg, Carbohydrates 20 g, Fiber 1 g, Sugars 9 g, Protein 2 g

Dietary Exchanges: 1½ other carbohydrate

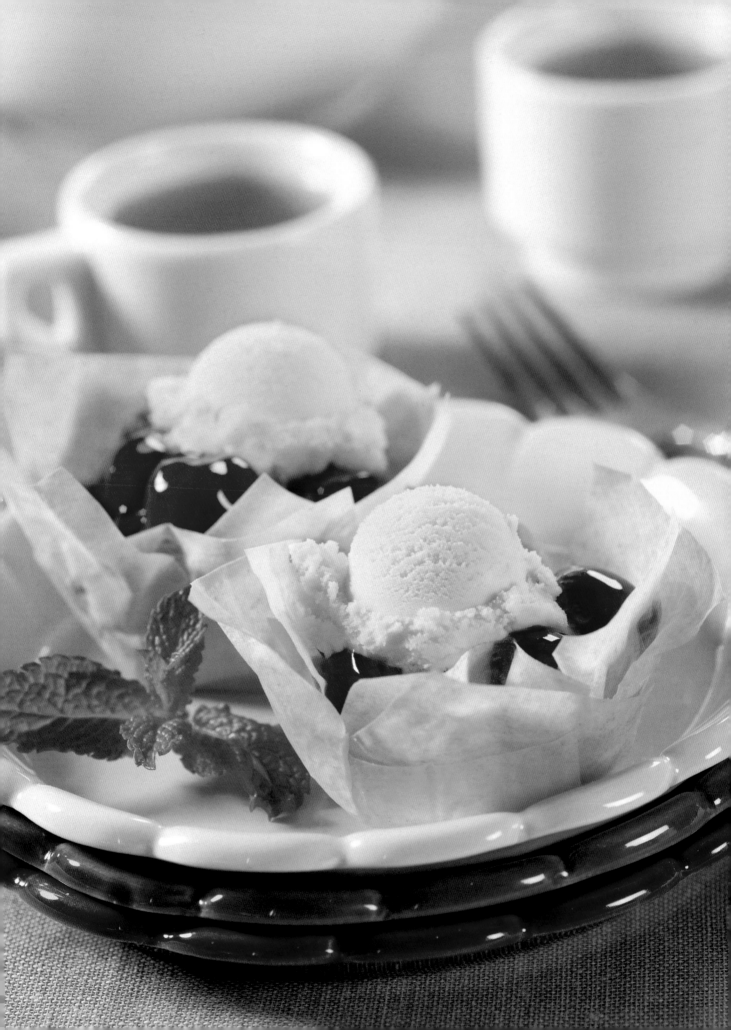

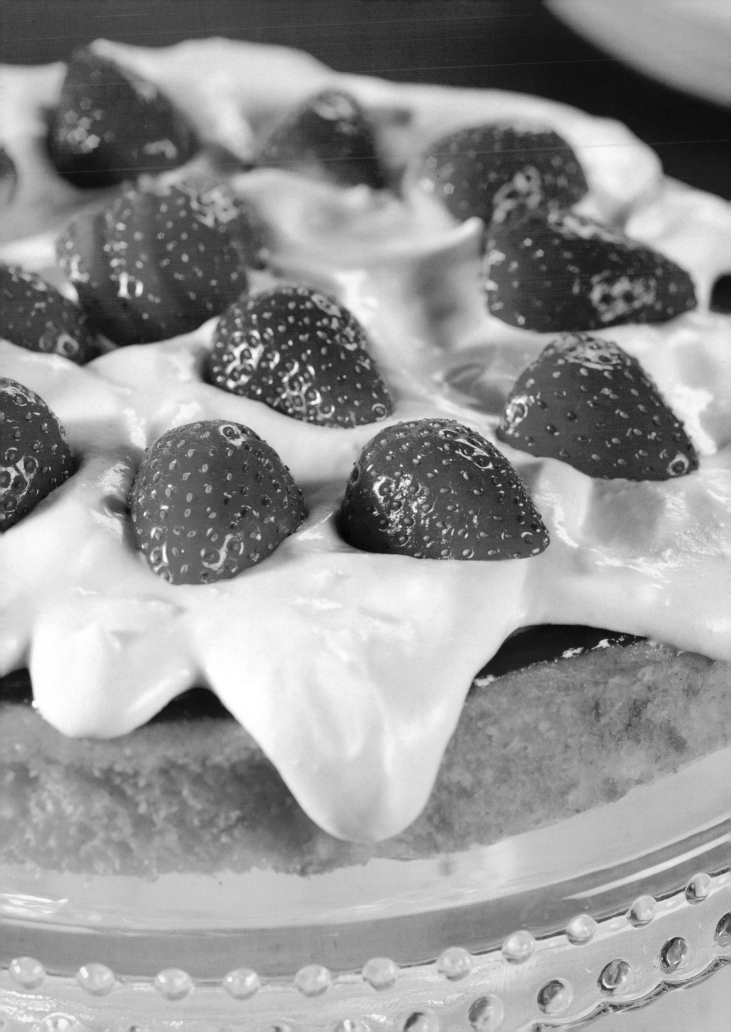

STRAWBERRY PUDDLE CAKE

SERVES 10; 1 slice per serving

Vegetable oil spray
1 9-ounce box single-layer yellow cake mix
Whites of 2 large eggs
1 teaspoon grated orange zest
½ cup fresh orange juice, divided
4 ounces fat-free or reduced-fat cream cheese, softened
1 cup thawed fat-free or light frozen whipped topping
1 cup marshmallow creme
3 tablespoons fat-free milk
½ cup raspberry all-fruit spread
1 teaspoon grated peeled gingerroot
2 cups whole strawberries (about 8 ounces), stems discarded, halved

Preheat the oven to 350°F. Lightly spray a 9-inch round cake pan with vegetable oil spray.

In a medium mixing bowl, beat the cake mix, egg whites, orange zest, and ¼ cup orange juice with an electric mixer on high speed for 2 minutes, scraping the side as needed. Pour in the remaining ¼ cup orange juice. Beat for 2 minutes. Pour into the cake pan.

Bake on the center rack for 20 minutes, or until a cake tester or wooden toothpick inserted in the center comes out clean. Place on a cooling rack. Let stand for 10 minutes. Invert onto a cake platter or plate. Let cool completely.

Meanwhile, in a medium mixing bowl, beat the cream cheese on low speed until smooth. Add the whipped topping, marshmallow creme, and milk, and mix on low speed until smooth.

In a small microwaveable bowl, stir together the fruit spread and gingerroot. Microwave on 50 percent power (medium) for 15 to 20 seconds, or until just melted. Whisk until smooth. If hot, let stand for 1 minute to cool. Pour the fruit sauce on the top of the cooled cake. Spread evenly over the top only; do not let the sauce drip down the side.

Pour the whipped topping mixture over the cake, letting the mixture flow down the side. Decoratively arrange the strawberry halves on top. Refrigerate for at least 2 hours, or until the icing is slightly firm.

To serve, cut into 10 wedges. Place the wedges on plates. Spoon the puddled icing over the cake.

Nutrients per Serving: Calories 231, Total Fat 2.5 g, Saturated Fat 1.0 g, Polyunsaturated Fat 0.0 g, Monounsaturated Fat 0.0 g, Cholesterol 2 mg, Sodium 242 mg, Carbohydrates 47 g, Fiber 1 g, Sugars 29 g, Protein 4 g
Dietary Exchanges: 3 other carbohydrate, ½ fat

CHERRY CHOCOLATE TIRAMISÙ

SERVES 8; 2×4-inch piece per serving

1 cup water

¼ cup sugar

2 teaspoons instant coffee granules

1 teaspoon vanilla extract

6 ounces ladyfingers, separated and torn into ½-inch pieces

8 ounces fat-free or light frozen whipped topping, thawed

2 tablespoons unsweetened cocoa powder

16 ounces frozen unsweetened pitted dark cherries, thawed, undrained

2 tablespoons sugar

1 tablespoon cornstarch

¼ teaspoon almond extract

¼ cup slivered almonds, dry-roasted

In a small bowl, stir together the water, ¼ cup sugar, coffee granules, and vanilla until the sugar has dissolved.

To assemble, place ½ of the ladyfinger pieces in an 8-inch square baking pan. Stir the coffee mixture and spoon half over the ladyfingers. Spoon ½ whipped topping over the ladyfingers, spreading evenly. Using a fine sieve, sprinkle ½ of the cocoa powder over all. Repeat. Cover with plastic wrap. Refrigerate for 8 to 24 hours.

Meanwhile, halve the cherries if desired. In a large skillet, stir together the cherries and their liquid, 2 tablespoons sugar, and cornstarch until the cornstarch is completely dissolved. Bring to a boil over medium-high heat. Boil for 1 minute, stirring constantly. (A flat spatula works well for this so you can scrape the bottom, where the mixture thickens first.) Remove from the heat.

Put the skillet on a cooling rack. Stir in the almond extract. Let the mixture cool completely, about 15 minutes. Refrigerate in a plastic resealable bag or airtight container until serving time.

To serve, spoon the cherry mixture over individual servings of tiramisù. Sprinkle with the almonds.

Nutrients per Serving: Calories 246, Total Fat 2.5 g, Saturated Fat 0.0 g, Polyunsaturated Fat 0.5 g, Monounsaturated Fat 1.0 g, Cholesterol 4 mg, Sodium 69 mg, Carbohydrates 51 g, Fiber 2 g, Sugars 32 g, Protein 3 g

Dietary Exchanges: 1 fruit, 2½ other carbohydrate, ½ fat

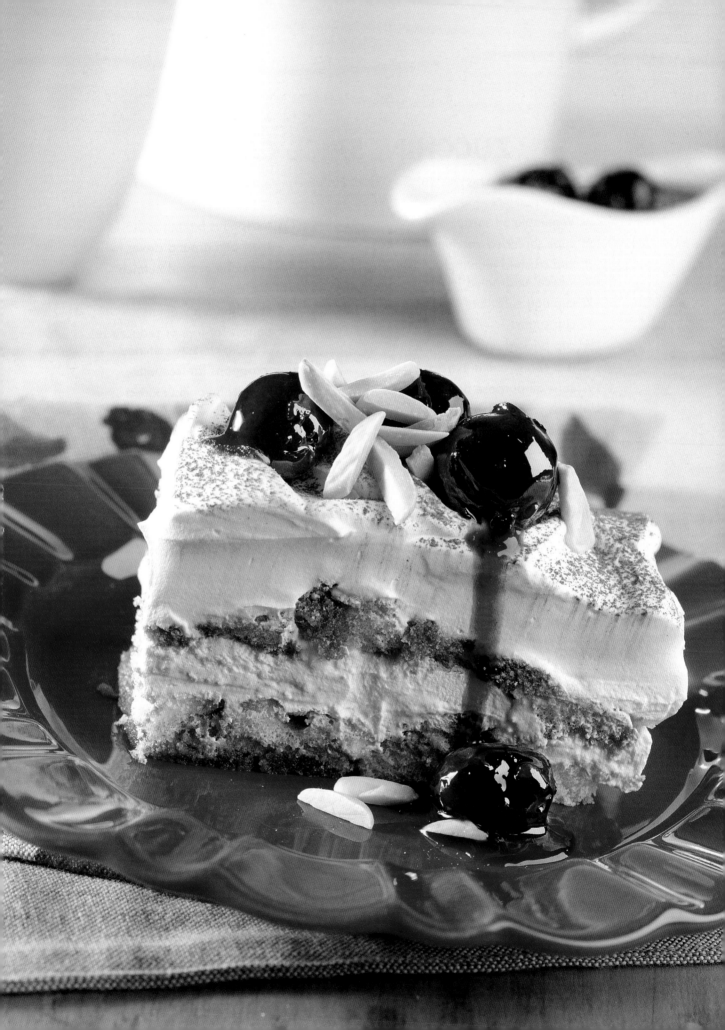

ZUCCHINI SPICE CAKE

SERVES 16; 3¼×2¼-inch piece per serving

Vegetable oil spray
2 cups shredded zucchini or carrots
1 cup crushed pineapple in its own juice, undrained
¾ cup egg substitute
¾ cup sugar
½ cup packed dark brown sugar
1 teaspoon vanilla extract
1¼ cups all-purpose flour
1¼ cups whole-wheat flour
1½ teaspoons ground cinnamon

1¼ teaspoons baking soda
1 teaspoon ground cloves
1 teaspoon ground nutmeg
¾ cup raisins
½ cup chopped walnuts
4 ounces fat-free or reduced-fat cream cheese, softened
1½ teaspoons fat-free milk
¾ teaspoon vanilla extract
2 cups unsifted confectioners' sugar

Preheat the oven to 350°F. Lightly spray a 13×9×2-inch glass baking dish with vegetable oil spray.

In a large bowl, stir together the zucchini, pineapple, egg substitute, sugars, and 1 teaspoon vanilla. Add the flours, cinnamon, baking soda, cloves, and nutmeg, stirring just to moisten and blend the dry ingredients. Fold in the raisins and walnuts. Spoon into the baking dish, smoothing the top. Bake for 45 to 50 minutes, or until a wooden toothpick or cake tester inserted in the center comes out clean. Let cool completely on a cooling rack.

Meanwhile, in a large mixing bowl, beat the cream cheese, milk, and ¾ teaspoon vanilla with an electric mixer on low until smooth. Add the confectioners' sugar 1 cup at a time, beating after each addition until smooth. Cover and refrigerate.

To serve, cut the servings needed and place on dessert plates. Drizzle with the glaze. Cover and refrigerate leftover cake without the glaze. Cover and refrigerate the glaze separately.

Nutrients per Serving: Calories 263, Total Fat 3.0 g, Saturated Fat 0.5 g, Polyunsaturated Fat 2.0 g, Monounsaturated Fat 0.5 g, Cholesterol 1 mg, Sodium 164 mg, Carbohydrates 56 g, Fiber 3 g, Sugars 38 g, Protein 6 g

Dietary Exchanges: 4 other carbohydrate, ½ fat

Recipe Index